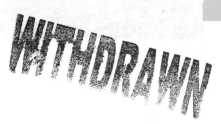

Core Curriculum for Reflexology in the United Kingdom

FIRST EDITION 2006

British Library - A CIP Catalogue
record for this book is available
from the British Library.

I.S.B.N.   0-9553122-8-0

Published by

Douglas Barry Publications

Kemp House
152 - 160 City Road
London
EC1V 2NX
ENGLAND

Tel 0870 879 3828
Fax 0870 879 2865

E-mail: info@DouglasBarry.com

1 CONTENTS/INDEX

Sections	Title	Page
1	Contents/Index	1
2	Introduction	2
3	Course content	6
4	**Theory, origin & development**	**8**
5	**Technique**	**17**
6	**Clinical Practice**	**26**
7	**Anatomy and Physiology**	**46**
8	**Relating Reflexology to Health**	**89**

Appendices

Appendix 1: Course		**94**
A1.1	Course Title	94
A1.2	Sector	95
A1.3	Course Hours and Duration	95
A1.4	Student Entry Requirements	97
A1.5	First Aid Requirement	98
A1.6	Course Teacher Qualifications	100
Appendix 2: Assessment		**101**
A2.1	Assessment Strategy	101
A2.2	Assessment Scheme	101
A2.3	Suitable Assessment Tools	102
A2.4	Mapping of Assessment Tools with Learning Outcomes	102
A2.5	Client Studies, Case Studies and External Treatment Practice	103
Appendix 3: Recommended reading and lists		**106**
A3.1	Reflexology Text Books	106
A3.2	Anatomy & Physiology/Human Biology Text Books	107
A3.3	Books related to Medicine – Conventional and CAM	108
A3.4	Other Useful, Interesting or Comparative texts	109
A3.5	Reflexology Forum Listed Foot (and Hand) Charts	111
A3.6	Contraindications and Cautions to be Exercised in Reflexology	112
Appendix 4: National Occupation Standards		**115**
A4.1	Mapping of Reflexology NOS against Core Curriculum	115
A4.2	Skills for Health Assessment Guidance	119
A4.3	Career Progression in Reflexology	124
Appendix 5: Current legislation		**125**
Appendix 6: Levels		**126**
A6.1	Training and Education Levels	126
A6.2	Vocational Levels	127
A6.3	The Recommended Level of this Core Curriculum	127
Appendix 7: Glossary of terms		**129**
Appendix 8: References		**131**

2 INTRODUCTION

The Reflexology Forum, as part of the Regulatory process for Reflexology, commissioned this Core Curriculum in July 2001. Recognising this to be a huge and unpaid task, volunteers were sought to form a Working Group. This group was to be made up of individuals representing the member organisations of the Reflexology Forum with the relevant experience and expertise. It is a credit to the individuals involved, and the members that no doubt supported them, that this document has been produced. It is also worthy of note that many of these contributors had previously spent many years donating their resources to the production of the National Occupational Standards, with which this curriculum is intended to work.

To reflect the entire range of Reflexology learning the name of the working group was changed from the 'Education Working Group' to the 'Education and Training Working Group' (the EaT group).

The Reflexology Forum and the Prince's Foundation for Integrated Health have funded the expense of holding a minimum of four group meetings per annum. The Working Group has reported back to the Forum at its quarterly meetings and will present this document in its draft form for acceptance by the entire Reflexology Forum before its general consultation release.

The Process adopted by the Education and Training Working Group in producing the Core Curriculum was:

1. To decide upon the Terms of Reference for the working group:
   - 'To take forward the work of the Reflexology Forum in respect of Education and Training in order to build on the Established National Occupational Standards for Reflexology.'
   - 'To develop an *over-arching core curriculum, methods of assessment and criteria for assessment of knowledge and competence*. These will be owned by the whole Reflexology Forum and in due course form the basis for a nationally recognised qualification.'

2. Produce an analytical report of the entire range of training provision in the UK in relation to these aspects:
   - Course Title
   - Linked Organisations
   - Awarding Body
   - Training Provider information
   - Sector/s involved
   - Level (e.g. NVQ 1–5 or Academic 1–3)
   - Minimum Course Duration
   - Teacher Contact Hours (now Guided Learning Hours) Home Study Hours, Examination Hours (if any)
   - Assessment Strategy

- Entry Requirements
- Teacher or Tutor/Assessor Qualifications Required
- Cost

In addition, information specific to Reflexology was collated:
- Case Study Requirement (if any)
- Contraindications Specified
- Insurance Conditions and any linked Insurers
- Mandatory current First Aid required
- If hands and ears were included as well as feet and
- Course content included, with specific regard to:
  - Theory
  - Technique
  - Clinical Practice
  - Anatomy and Physiology and
  - Pathology (knowledge of commonly encountered conditions and disorders)

3. From the report above it was possible to decide upon the current need to improve the general standard of the data in the first column above and recommendations were made to the Forum on 29th May 2002.

4. A policy of 'tasking' was adopted to share the considerable volume of work in analysing column two above. At one EaT meeting projects were allocated to individuals or sub groups who then worked on this during the period before the next meeting when they reported back. This considerably reduced the meeting load to planning and refinements and eliminated the carousel of needless group debate.

5. A 'Commonality Exercise' questionnaire was devised by the chair and distributed to participating organisation representatives. To bolster the spirit of cooperation and inclusiveness that continues to pervade the Reflexology Forum the emphasis of the questioning was to underline the *similarities* between different reflexology methodologies and let this then highlight differences. The collated results of this project informed the course content. This was encouraging in that the suspected wide variation in existing education and training was less than the commonalities.

6. The 'core' aspect of the curriculum was helpful in determining that much of the wide range of reflexology techniques can be removed from the 'core' and included in specialist training packages delivered as CPD modules. What has been called 'Pure' or 'Classical' reflexology can be classified as two definable, slightly different techniques that it is possible to deliver either independently or in combination with the approval of the entire EaT group.

7. When the results of the sub group 'tasks' were received and compiled it was a relatively simple, although time-consuming, project to compile the information into this document.

8. **Second Draft:** Between September 2003 and September 2004 the first draft of this document was distributed to the participating organisations within the Reflexology Forum who, in turn, selected individuals/training providers to scrutinise the format and contents and respond with their comments and suggestions. (Although attempt has been made to thank these responders individually, it is appropriate here to thank all individuals who have given freely many hours of their time to provide the many replies received. Many of these suggestions we have been able to accommodate, in whole, or part, into this second draft.)

9. In addition to Forum members the first draft was sent to other interested parties such as the Prince's Foundation for Integrated Health, Skills for Health, several awarding bodies with an interest in Reflexology and reflexology organisations not yet Forum members.

10. During the year of producing the second draft there were personnel changes to the EaT group, which positively changed the dynamics of the team. The original members being experts in the delivering of Reflexology enabled the curriculum content to be comprehensive. The later addition of some educationally qualified and experienced team members then provided the needed expertise to develop the delivery details of the curriculum.

Statement of Need

As highlighted in the report referred to in 2 above, a prime requirement of this curriculum was to bring to reflexology education and training provision in the UK a common foundation that would end the disparity in course content and depth and provide a thread of continuity between practitioners that could be recognised by, and thus reassure, the public. This will work to ensure the safety and effectiveness of graduates and provide a minimum standard of learning and skill upon which the rich variety and diversity of the individual practitioners can then be built.

To provide a minimum foundation for all practitioners it has been necessary to return to the roots of reflexology and decide upon a core training that can provide elements recognisable to clients, regardless of where their practitioner was taught. To achieve this it has been necessary to be quite prescriptive in this document to ensure commonality. It will also explain the leaning toward a factual, scientific and medical approach. Reflexology is holistic in its approach but this does not conflict with gaining understanding, and developing the science, of how it works. Reflexology is also a healing art which can be cultivated on a bed of knowledge and fact. The wealth of variety of the talents that different practitioners and tutors bring to the profession can still flourish on this core curriculum. As reflexology is now offered as standard treatment in hospital, hospice and private medical institutions and integrated health is now a reality, there is no apology for a medical approach. Clients openly seek help with health problems and conventional medicine openly seeks help from complementary medicine with symptom control and more.

It is appropriate at this point to thank, alphabetically, the following whose contributions to this document have been essential:

Mark Baker	(Association of Reflexologists)
Carol Bailey	(Independent Chair, Reflexology Forum)
Beryl Crane	(Reflexologists Society)
Hildegard Edwards	(International Institute of Reflexology, UK)
Miriam Evans	(Professional Association of Clinical Therapists)
Geraldine Giles	(Association of Reflexologists)
Heather Gillette	(Association of Reflexologists)
Irene Gunn	(International Institute of Reflexology, UK)
Nicola Hall	(British Reflexology Association)
John Hopson	(Reflexologists Society)
Carol Jamison	(International Institute of Reflexology, UK)
Ann Lett	(British School of Reflex Zone Therapy)
Jennie Levick	(International Institute of Reflexology, UK)
Lynne Marland	(Centre for Clinical Reflexology)
Heather Mole	(Vocational Training Charitable Trust)
Ann Noblett	(Guild of Complementary Practitioners)
Margaret Smillie	(Scottish Institute of Reflexologists)
Susan Stirling	(International Guild of Professional Practitioners)
Renée Tanner	(International Federation of Reflexologists)
Pat Turton	(University of West England)
Julia Williams	(Complementary Therapies Association)

Appreciation for consultative support must be given to:

Tom Lane	(Skills for Health)
Hazel Russo	(Foundation for Integrated Health)
Lorraine Williams	(Foundation for Integrated Health)

Clive S. O'Hara
Chair, Reflexology Forum Education and Training Working Group

3 COURSE CONTENT

3.1 Overview

The course content is divided into five components of subject knowledge, all of which have both practical and theoretical aspects requiring assessment to demonstrate skill and competence and examination to test knowledge and understanding. The components are:

Section	Component
4	Theory, Origin and Development
5	Technique
6	Clinical Practice
7	Anatomy and Physiology
8	Relating Reflexology to Health

The sequence in which these components are covered in a course is not important, except where specifically referred to in the course notes. We would strongly recommend the use of a workbook requiring completion by the student of assignments, exercises, questions, tables and diagrams which can be continually assessed and when finished will evidence full coverage of that content. The presentation and layout of the question paper can be of similar format to the workbook, and this will aid recall for the student during examination.

3.2 Content Extent and Limitation

The wording of the content is designed to show the extent end limit of the knowledge and understanding of each aspect of the component that the Reflexology Forum specifies.

For example, in Anatomy and Physiology during coursework a student may be required to complete the names of the bones on a drawing of the skeleton. However, an examination paper would require the names of the individual bones of the foot and hand but not the entire body. The names of the bones required will be found in the subject content and merely awareness of the rest will be sufficient.

3.2.1 Naming of Reflex Points

As the location of reflexes is integral to the concept of reflexology, the location of these onto an unlabelled diagram could be an exception to the general rule of not having students draw diagrams from memory. The entire list of reflexes to be located and identified is in the content.

3.2.2 Differences in Charts

Tolerance to the difference between reflexology charts or 'maps' is built into the content. A list of charts currently acceptable to the Reflexology Forum can be found in the Recommended Reading List. In due course the Reflexology Forum will have to address the resolving of chart differences, but in the meantime students will benefit from being shown how to assess the accuracy of reflex areas in practice, and will settle down with which one from the list they are comfortable.

3.3 Content Extent and Limitation

3.3.1 Knowledge of Disorders & Disease: 'Relating Reflexology to Health'

A list of diseases and disorders is included in course content Section 8 and an example of a workbook entry is also included here. The knowledge of ill health will be a definition of the disorder, observable symptoms, the usual causes and how it is usually treated by conventional medicine. It will then be related to reflexology by stating the reflex areas that would be most useful to emphasise during treatment, and the rationale for so doing along with any adaptation of the treatment that may be required to effectively cope with this client.

3.3.2 Client or Patient?

The issue of what to call those who receive reflexology is still open to debate and some practitioners hold very strong views. Some feel the word patient is too medical, while others feel 'client' places the emphasis on commercial interest rather than health.

A recent review of cancer patients surprisingly revealed that they felt very strongly that they should still be referred to as 'patients'. They suggested 'patient' positively implies healing and being cared for. Some authorities state that 'patient' negatively implies 'belonging to a doctor' (CRN 2005). However, as the unfriendly term 'service user' is also an authority suggestion, it is wise to ask the reflexology recipients what they would like to be called.

At a meeting of the Reflexology Forum Education and Training Group in 2004 a decision was made to use the word 'client' in the text of this curriculum document to refer to anyone who receives reflexology from a practitioner. 'Client' is thus here used to cover the word 'patient' even if that is how they are referred to in their environment – for example on a hospital ward or in a hospice.

3.4 Learning Outcomes – Wording and Presentation

The following sections of this curriculum document, 4–8, contain the five course content components. Each section has a brief overview of the component followed by the learning outcome statements for that section. The specific verbs for each statement are italicised. Immediately following the leaning outcomes is a table of these verbs mapped against the range of suitable assessment tools from Appendix 2, to enable training providers and assessors to plan their programme to encompass all facets of the section.

4 THEORY, ORIGIN & DEVELOPMENT

Recommended Teacher Contact Hours – **30**	Expected Home Study Hours – **100**

MAIN OBJECTIVES

Section 4 of this curriculum deals with the theoretical aspects of reflexology, its history, and development from ancient times down to the twentieth century formation of what is practised today. Current hypotheses as to how reflexology works are covered along with the underpinning knowledge of where the reflex points and areas are located on the feet, and later, the hands. The *limitations* to what comes under the umbrella of reflexology are outlined and many areas considered by some to be reflexology are put outside the curriculum in the interests of standardisation. The student is encouraged to consider these via CPD after cultivating a solid foundation in 'pure' reflexology, which stands alone as a complete complementary medical practice at practitioner level. The *extent* to which this curriculum reaches is a project to develop a particular reflexology concept. This, preferably run during the second year, has the wide objective to stimulate research awareness and develop research or audit skills. This aspect is especially vital to reflexology, which is in urgent need of published robust evidence.

LEARNING OUTCOMES FOR SECTION 4

After completing this section of the curriculum a student will be able to:

4.1   *State* a concise definition reflexology to demonstrate their own understanding and accurately inform prospective clients.

4.2   *Demonstrate* knowledge of, and *evaluate* the significance of, the ancient origins of reflexology from the apparent earliest reference in Egypt and then other parts of the world until 1900.

4.3   *Demonstrate* knowledge of the modern day development of reflexology from Zone Therapy.

4.3.1   *State* the principle of Zone Theory, *name* and precisely *locate* 4 lateral zones on a blank diagram.
State what cross reflexes or referral areas are, *name* seven pairs and *evaluate* their significance to reflexology.

4.3.2   *Evaluate* the relevance of Eunice Ingham's contribution and *state* how she developed zone theory into reflexology.
Demonstrate knowledge of Hanne Marquardt's role and the difference between reflexology and Reflex Zone Therapy.

4.3.3   *Evaluate* the importance of the early UK reflexology pioneers, *name 3 (three)* and *be able to trace and map* their own line of training.

4.4   *Name* and *demonstrate* knowledge of the roles of the bodies and organisations concerned with reflexology in the UK.

4.5 *Demonstrate* an understanding of the main current hypotheses as to how reflexology works and *evaluate* their usefulness.

4.5.1 *Demonstrate* an understanding of the effect of the therapeutic relationship; the © 'reflexology package'; placebo and relaxation.

4.5.2 *State* the meaning of the terms Holism, Complementary Medicine, Alternative Medicine and CAM.

4.5.3 *Recognise* that some subject areas and treatment systems are outside this curriculum which is solely concerned with training to be a practitioner of reflexology.

4.6 *Demonstrate* an understanding of the variety of reflexology 'maps' or charts and *analyse* the various charts with a view to choosing accurate location of reflex points and areas.

4.6.2 *Recall* and *locate* on a blank diagram of a foot, and later a hand, all 73 reflex points and areas listed in Table 4.6.2. *Recall* and *locate* on a blank diagram of a foot, and later a hand, 4 transverse guidelines and the vertical tendon guide line.

4.7 *Design, manage,* and *evaluate* a research based or audit type of project related to reflexology OR *critique* an existing published piece of reflexology research.

4.8 *Demonstrate* an understanding of a treatment pattern.
Analyse the method of treating right and left feet (and hands) separately contrasted with treating both sides simultaneously, *evaluate* the benefits and *synthesise* a treatment sequence to be used as a basis for effective and consistent treatment.

LEARNING OUTCOMES MAPPED AGAINST ASSESSMENT TOOLS
(See Appendix 2)

Tool	Learning Outcome Verbs
Case Studies	analyse; demonstrate; discuss; explain;
Client Studies	evaluate; list;
Home Treatments	evaluate; list; locate
Blank Feet/Hand Diagrams to locate Reflex Points/Areas	draw; locate; recall;
Blank Diagrams of Body Parts to Labels A&P Items	draw; locate; recall;
2000 to 5000-word Assignments At level 2 At level 3	analyse; assess; analyse; assess; critique, evaluate; synthesise;
Interim (Formative) Assessments (Written)	draw; locate; recall;
Interim (Formative) Assessments (Practical)	articulate, demonstrate; demonstrate understanding;
Final (Summative) Assessments (Written)	draw; locate; recall;
Final (Summative) Assessments (Practical)	demonstrate;
Professional Portfolio	analyse, articulate, list,
Interview	articulate, explain; list; recall; state;
Project: Research based or audit	analyse, design, evaluate, manage,

COURSE CONTENT

4.1 Definition of Reflexology

Students should *develop* from the outset a concise definition with which they are comfortable, but including essential key phrases synonymous with:

- 'reflex points and areas in the hands & feet';
- 'relating to corresponding body parts';
- 'precise hand & finger pressure techniques';
- 'normalization, homeostasis, or balance';
- 'improving circulation';
- 'relaxation' or 'stress relief';
- 'helping the body to heal itself 'or 'activating the body's healing processes'; and
- 'prevention'.

An example of a concise definition could be:

'Reflexology is the study and practice of treating reflex points and areas in the feet and hands that relate to corresponding parts of the body. Using precise hand and finger techniques a reflexologist can improve circulation, induce relaxation and enable homeostasis. These three outcomes can activate the body's own healing systems to heal and prevent ill health.'

4.2 Ancient Origins of Reflexology

The student should be able to *appreciate* the balanced significance of ancient Egypt as the earliest evidence of what appears to be 'reflexology'. (Understanding of the tomb wall relief and translation should be included.) Students should also be *aware* of the evidence of similar practice in areas including China, the Far East, India, North America, Europe and Africa.

4.3 Modern Day Development

4.3.1 Zone Theory

Appreciation of the roles played by Sir Henry Head, Sir Charles Sherrington, Dr William Fitzgerald, Joe Shelby (Selby) Riley, Edwin Bowers should be included in content. Joseph Corvo should be noted as being the main proponent for zone therapy in the UK.

10 Zones

The student should be able to *state* the premise of Zone Theory:

The human body can be divided into 10 longitudinal zones and 'constant, direct pressure upon any part of a particular zone can have an anaesthetising effect on another part of that same zone'.

Kunz & Kunz, 1984

Transverse Zones or Guide Lines

The student should *know* that guide lines or transverse zones were later added and be able to *name* and *precisely locate* these:

Shoulder, diaphragm, waist and pelvic floor/heel line.

Students should *know* the precise location of the Flexor Hallucis Longus or Plantar Tendon and *appreciate* its importance as a Guideline.

Cross Reflexes or Referral Areas

Students should also *understand* the nature of cross reflexes/referral areas/zone related areas; be able to *name* seven pairs (below); and *understand* when and how to integrate the knowledge of this relationship into reflexology practice:

For example, the fact that hands can be used to deliver reflexology depends on the fact that they are referral areas to the feet.

Hip	Thigh	Knee	Lower leg	Ankle	Foot	Toes
Shoulder	Upper arm	Elbow	Forearm	Wrist	Hand	Fingers

4.3.2 Zone Therapy into Reflexology

Eunice Ingham

Students must be able to *evaluate* the importance of the work of Eunice Ingham as the original pioneer of reflexology, and should be able to explain the three major transitions she established to build reflexology from zone therapy:

1. She identified the feet as a target for attention due to their position at the base of the longitudinal zones;
2. charted or 'mapped' the feet in detail locating the original 'reflexes', and;
3. added the technique of 'variable and alternating pressure' to the previous zone therapy method of 'constant direct pressure'.

Hanne Marquardt

Students should also be able to *recall* the role Hanne Marquardt has played in the development of Reflex Zone Therapy and the similarities and differences of the disciplines.

4.3.3 Reflexology and the UK

Doreen Bayly

Students should also be able to *evaluate* the role Doreen Bayly has played in bringing Reflexology to the UK

UK 'Pioneers'

The student must appreciate the importance of the role played by the early 'pioneers' of bringing reflexology into the UK and be aware of the subtle differences in philosophy and technique that have resulted from the constraints of early training methods.

'Family Tree'

With the help of their tutor each student should be encouraged to *trace* their reflexology 'family tree' to establish the line through which their training developed.

Significant UK developers

[The Core Curriculum Working group decided that the criteria for inclusion in this list is – 'being actively involved in developing reflexology and delivering treatments for more than 25 years prior to Jan 2006' and seeks nominations for such significant individuals.]

4.4 UK Bodies & Organisations

Bodies & Organisations

Students should be made aware of the existence of bodies, associations and organisations currently concerned with reflexology in the UK. They should also understand the acronyms, roles and areas of focus of these: Reflexology Forum (RF) and its member organisations; Prince's Foundation for Integrated Health (PFIH); Skills for Health (SfH); Qualifications and Curriculum Agency (QCA); the Institute for Complementary Medicine (ICM) and the British Complementary Medicine Association (BCMA).

NOS & reports

Students should be aware of the early significance of the NOS (first published 1998; republished 2001 by Healthworks UK); the House of Lords' 6th Report on CAM (2001); the FIM report (1995) and the Exeter report (2000) in the development of the standards for CAM.

Students should be able to explain the difference between statutory and voluntary regulation and be aware of how they personally and currently stand with regard to regulation

4.5 Current Theory and Scientific Understanding

4.5.1 Theories

Students should be aware of the fact that none of the current theories of how reflexology works have been established as fact and are still the subject of debate. However, they should be aware of the probable significance to reflexology of the following hypotheses:

Hypothesis	References
Pain gate control	Melzack & Wall, 1965
Nerve impulse theory	Bliss & Bliss, 2000
Electromagnetic theories	eg Bliss & Bliss, 1999
Energy blockage theories	Kunz & Kunz, 1985
or lactic acid theory/'U bend' theory	Bliss & Bliss, 1999
Endorphin/encephalin release theory	Ginsberg & Famey, 1987
Autonomic & somatic integration theory	Kunz & Kunz, 1998
Proprioceptive theory	Kunz & Kunz, 1988
Meridian theory	Dougans 1996, Crane 1996

Embryo containing information of the   Frandsen, 1998
whole organism (ECIWO) theory

Other Theoretical Input

Students should also be able to evaluate the relevance of the *Placebo effect*. The effect of the *Therapeutic Relationship* (NOS, 2001) between client and practitioner and the overall effect of © *'the Reflexology Package'* (e.g. Mackereth & Tiran, 2000) should also be covered in the course content. The power of the effect of *relaxation* upon a client without other interventions should not be excluded.

4.5.2 Attendant Philosophies

The student should also be able to *restate* the meaning of the terms Holism and Complementary Medicine and relate these to reflexology. The meanings of the term Alternative Medicine and the acronym CAM should also be *known*.

4.5.3 Exclusions

Whilst considered by some to be important to reflexology, the following subject areas should be considered as separate philosophies and so would not be part of a reflexology course content:

The aura and chakras; colour therapy; use of crystals and dowsing during reflexology; meridians.

There are many treatment programmes, some incorporating the word reflex or reflexology that can be considered extensions or additions to, developments of, deviations from and adaptations of, 'classical' 'standard' or 'pure' reflexology and thus would not be part of a reflexology practitioner course. Some add techniques and concepts to those included in this curriculum, others may incorporate a small part of the curriculum content into another therapy. A student wishing to study these would do so through additional training. This additional training could be via CPD and inclusion on a future Reflexology Forum CPD list could indicate recognition.

It is important that to merit the designation 'Reflexologist' the minimum training is the entire content of this curriculum. Once they have achieved Reflexology Practitioner status a person can obtain insurance and practice autonomously without a need to diversify.

It may be that some providers will offer practitioner training incorporating such a speciality. Such providers and their students should ensure the entire core curriculum is included during such training to achieve practitioner status.

4.5.4 CPD

Although this curriculum is complete in the education and training of a Reflexology Practitioner, graduates have a responsibility to continually develop their profession (CPD), refine their skill and update their knowledge. This is not the same as the option of embarking on courses in different styles of reflexology.

4.6 Location of Reflex Points/Areas

4.6.1 Knowledge or Skill?

Although the working of reflex points/areas is a practical skill and can be assessed as such via performance criteria, the reasoning behind the location of each is academic/knowledge based. Such subject content is reasonably placed under this heading of reflexology theory and development. The aspect of development is connected with the variety and differences in foot (and hand) charts/maps and requires the student to *analyse* information. In addition to the analysis of existing reflex points/areas the ongoing progression of reflexology theory requires *research* and the *synthesis* of fresh information.

Level 4 status

The above can argue for a vocational level 4 and an academic diploma level (2) status for this practitioner course. Modules at academic degree level (3) already exist.

'Degree'/Academic Level 3

Reflexology courses are already offered at universities across the UK in modular form set at academic levels 2 (diploma) and 3 (degree). As the location of reflex points is currently a mixture of theoretical placement and empirical evidence there is a need to encourage robust research if reflexology is to achieve full integration into mainstream healthcare. Including core content that encourages research, evaluation and synthesis will further establish the need for level 4.

4.6.2 List of Reflex Points/Areas

The list of reflex points and areas that follows has been compiled from a collection of charts from reputable sources (see Appendix 2). Course tutors and students should be encouraged to *be inclusive in their awareness of charts* and where differences and slight variations occur *seek to establish commonality* through practice on clients with known problems. Future research should ensure more consistency in mapping reflex points and areas onto charts.

Table 4.6.2: Reflex Points/Areas to be Located

Adrenal Glands
Anus
Appendix
Arm
Axillary lymphatics
Back – Upper, Mid & Lower
Bladder
Brain
Breast (especially female)
Bronchial Tubes
Buttocks
Coeliac ganglion (Solar Plexus)
Colon
Diaphragm
Duodenum
Ears – *along ridge under toes 3–5; up toes 3–4, on hallux*
Elbow
Eustachian tube
Eyes – *along ridge under toes 2–3; on toes 2–3, on hallux*
Face
Fallopian (Uterine) Tubes
Gall Bladder
Groin
Head
Heart
Hepatic Flexure
Hip
Hypothalamus
Ileocaecal 'Valve'
Inguinal lymphatics
Jaw
Kidneys
Knee
Larynx/Pharynx
Leg
Liver
Lungs
Lymphatic duct
Lymphatic 'valleys'
Mammary lymphatics

Mouth/Tongue
Neck & Throat
Nose
Oesophagus
Ovary/Testicle
Pancreas
Pelvic Area
Pineal gland
Pituitary Gland
Pyloric Sphincter
Rectum
Ribs
Sacro-iliac joint
Sciatic areas
Shoulders
Sinuses
Small Intestines
Solar Plexus
Spine: Atlas & axis, Cervical, Thoracic, Lumbar, Sacrum & Coccyx
Spleen
Splenic flexure
Sternum
Stomach
Teeth
Thyroid, Parathyroid
Thoracic duct
Thymus
Tonsils/adenoids
Ureters
Uterus/Prostate
Wrists

Transverse Guide Lines
Shoulder Line
Diaphragm Line
Waistline
Pelvic/Heel Line

Vertical Guide Line
Tendon Line (Flexor Hallucis Longus)

Note: The Reflex points/areas above are listed alphabetically and not in any significant order, sequence or priority. During training the complete list of reflex points should be covered.

4.7 'Research' Project

For the course to be at an academic level that merits Practitioner status, and for the development of reflexology to be accepted as a medical science and achieve full integration, it is suggested that a research element be built into the content.

This would not have to be subjected to the full rigours of a research trial as would be required for a PhD. However, a way of demonstrating the analytical and evaluative skills of academic level 2, and the synthesis of academic level 3, which both match vocational national level 4, would be to design a research type project, or carry out an audit.

Some training courses have already been incorporating this element and much useful data has already been collected by this encouragement to students to carry out research type projects, and some suggestions for subjects that could be useful for trial are listed here:

- The effect of reflexology on easily measurable data e.g.:
    - Blood pressure
    - Blood glucose levels on diabetic clients
- The effect of reflexology upon people with specific illness/symptoms such as:
    - Migraine
    - Multiple Sclerosis
    - Stress
    - Fertility

Clinical Practice also lends itself to research subjects or audit projects:
- Is there an optimum time between treatments?

Are more frequent short treatments better than less frequent and longer treatments?
- Is treating both feet together better than completing one foot first before working the other? Left or right foot first?

Non-clinical subjects can also be appropriate for helping students see the importance of research:
- Which is the most suitable working medium?
- Which is the most suitable portable/static couch?

4.8 Treatment Pattern

A number of treatment patterns exists. The original approach to treatment was to treat first the Right Foot and then the Left Foot. However, some may now follow a sequence where the Left Foot is treated first, then the Right or others treat the body via systems involving both working both feet together. The pattern will be dependent on the training school method being taught.

All treatment patterns or sequences will involve treatment to ALL reflex points and areas of the feet. See **4.6.2** and **6.5.5**.

5 TECHNIQUE

Recommended Teacher Contact Hours – **50**   Expected Home Study Hours – **50**

REFLEXOLOGY TECHNIQUE

The practical aspects of executing reflexology extend to performing the following aspects of technique:

- *Relaxation routines* prior to, during and following the working of reflex points and areas
- The use of the *support hand* to facilitate effective treatment
- The application of various *pressure techniques* to effectively work different types of reflex points and areas
- The possible use of a medium to maintain a suitable texture for the effective application of technique
- The correct positioning of client and posture of practitioner to ensure efficient application of technique, comfort and safety

Assessment Strategy

Reflexology demands practical skill and will be continually assessed, formatively and summatively, throughout the course schedule. Toward the end of the course, a complete treatment with all its facets must be practically assessed. Consultation and client assessment, creating a therapeutic and hygienic environment, reflexology delivery technique, interpersonal skills, relating reflexes to the client's health, evaluating the treatment with the client, agreeing a treatment plan and treatment recording, must all be assessed, though it may only be viable for some training providers to accomplish this over several sessions (Section 7).

However, for this course to be set at its correct level (Section 6) and practitioner level, there is opportunity to demonstrate analytical and evaluative skills in the theory underpinning the various techniques, and questions will be set to test this knowledge and understanding during the final written assessment/examination.

Names of Techniques

As described in the theory, origin and development section there were many individual, charismatic pioneers responsible for the spread of reflexology during the mid 20th century and each has left their mark on technique. This has led to different names being applied to types of reflexology and relaxation techniques and variations in the style of performing these.

The Reflexology Forum has endeavoured to encompass these variations without dictating a rigid format, realising that where different terms are applied to similar movements these can be brought together. Following the lead set by the Prince of Wales's Foundation for Integrated Health, the spirit of cooperation that has fuelled the unification which helped the Reflexology Forum succeed is mirrored in this course content.

LEARNING OUTCOMES FOR SECTION 5

After completing this section of the curriculum a student will be able to:

5.1 *Demonstrate* the delivery and an *understanding* of **Foot Reflexology.** *Demonstrate* a minimum of six appropriate **relaxation techniques** from Table 5A and be able to *analyse* why some of these are best applied prior to working reflex points, interspersed throughout the treatment and at the conclusion of a reflexology session.

5.2 *Demonstrate* the appropriate use of the **support/holding hand** throughout the treatment, be able to *state* all the five functions of the holding hand and *evaluate* the importance of these five functions with relation to effective technique, client comfort and the practitioner's own health and safety.

5.3 *Demonstrate* the complete range of **reflexology pressure techniques** needed to effectively and safely work every reflex area listed in section 4.6.2 (table of reflex points and areas to be located) and be able to *state* which technique would be appropriate for which reflex when asked. Students will be able to demonstrate techniques from each section A, B, C, D of Table 5B though not asked to demonstrate the entire range.

5.4 *Demonstrate* a working knowledge of **appropriate mediums** to apply to the client's skin to achieve a texture enabling effective technique and be able to *explain* why they have chosen a particular medium, or none, for that treatment.

5.5 *Demonstrate* the correct **positioning** of their client/patient, be able to *defend* why support of their head, back, arms, backs of knees, legs and feet is appropriate and *analyse* how this relates to client comfort, health and safety, effective treatment and communication between client and practitioner.

5.5.1 *Demonstrate* the correct **positioning** of themselves whilst delivering reflexology treatment, be able to *state* how they should support their back and position their hands, arms, legs and feet and *analyse* how this relates to their own comfort, health and safety, effective treatment and communication between client and practitioner

5.5.2 *State* why it should be possible and preferable that the entire treatment is delivered with the practitioner seated.

5.6 *Demonstrate* the delivery and an understanding of **Hand reflexology** and *state* how the principle of referral areas/cross reflexes relates equally to reflexology on the hands as it does to the feet.

5.6.1 *Demonstrate* a minimum of six appropriate relaxation techniques from Table 5C and be able to *analyse* when some of these are best applied.

5.6.2 *Demonstrate* the appropriate use of the **support/holding hand** throughout the hand treatment and be able to *state* all the five functions of the support hand.

5.6.3 *Demonstrate* the complete range of reflexology **pressure techniques** needed to effectively and safely work every reflex area in the hands. Students will be able to demonstrate techniques from each section A, B, C, D of Table 5B, though not asked to demonstrate the entire range.

5.6.4   *Demonstrate* a working knowledge of **appropriate mediums** to apply to the client's hands to achieve a texture enabling effective technique and be able to *explain* why they have chosen a particular medium, or none, for that treatment.

5.6.5   *Demonstrate* the correct **positioning** of their client/patient for hand reflexology (refer to 5.5.2).

5.6.6   *Demonstrate* how set up their own treatment position during hand reflexology to prevent short-term discomfort and long-term damage.

LEARNING OUTCOMES MAPPED AGAINST ASSESSMENT TOOLS
(See Appendix 2)

Tool	Learning Outcome Verbs
Case Studies	analyse; demonstrate; discuss; explain;
Client Studies	evaluate; list;
Home Treatments	evaluate; list; locate
Blank Feet/Hand Diagrams to locate Reflex Points/Areas	draw; locate; recall;
Blank Diagrams of Body Parts to Labels A&P Items	draw; locate; recall;

2000 to 5000-word Assignments
    At level 2
    At level 3
	analyse; assess;
	analyse; assess; critique, evaluate; synthesise;

Interim (Formative) Assessments (Written)	draw; locate; recall;
Interim (Formative) Assessments (Practical)	articulate, demonstrate; demonstrate understanding;
Final (Summative) Assessments (Written)	draw; locate; recall;
Final (Summative) Assessments (Practical)	demonstrate;
Professional Portfolio	analyse, articulate, list,
Interview	articulate, explain; list; recall; state;
Project: Research based or audit	analyse, design, evaluate, manage,

COURSE CONTENT FOR SECTION 5

5.1 Relaxation Techniques

The student will be required to *demonstrate* a minimum of six appropriate relaxation techniques and be able to *analyse* why some of these are best applied *prior to* working reflex points, should be *interspersed throughout* the treatment and again *at the conclusion of* a reflexology session.

Foot Massage

Reflexology is often referred to as massage, which does not accurately describe the processes involved and their effect upon the client. Many of the relaxation techniques in Table 5A are related to massage. The techniques in Table 5B are not related to massage.

The student will not be expected to perform a *foot massage* before and/or after a treatment but use the relaxation techniques listed.

Table 5a is a compilation of commonly used relaxation techniques that can form a core list to which other techniques may be added as they are developed and evaluated during clinical practice.

If practitioners from diverse training backgrounds continue to use this common core of techniques it will present to the public a standardised treatment practice that has recognisable features. This can be reassuring to clients as they experience treatment with a familiar feel when visiting different practitioners.

As with pressure techniques tutors should emphasise the need to assess the needs of the client in relation to pressure and vigour when delivering all relaxation techniques. Students need to develop tactile and touch skills from the first day of training.

Table 5A: Relaxation Techniques

	Description	Name 1	Name 2
1	Gently place one palm on each plantar surface of the foot with as much surface contact as possible. Hold for up to 30 seconds. Used to initiate client contact	Palming	'Greeting the feet'
2	With one palm on each plantar surface perform a plantarflexion once, slide palms to perform a single dorsiflexion, then evert and invert the feet once. Used to ascertain mobility, detect resistance and encourage immediate relaxation. Use this immediately following 1 above and prior to ankle rotation	Stretching	Dorsiflexion Plantarflexion Eversion Inversion
3	Support the metatarsals between thumb and fingers of one hand and rest the heel of the foot with the other. Rotate the foot and ankle slowly several times in each direction	Ankle Rotation	Circumduction
4	With thumbs always adjacent, both hands encircle one foot from the medial aspect. The hand nearer the toes moves the foot forward and back. Make several twists progressing upward as though twisting the entire length of the spine reflex	Spinal Twist	Foot Wringing
5	Place both palms on either edge of the foot just below the toes. Keeping contact with foot, move the hands from side to side rapidly to loosen the foot. Keep the heel in contact with the couch to act as a pivot.	Side to Side	
6	Alternating pressure is applied by the flat fist to the upper plantar area whilst other hand cradles the opposite dorsal aspect to spread the metatarsals	Metatarsal Spread	Lung Press
7	Support the base of each toe with one hand and with the other holding near the base slowly rotate the toe with a gentle upward pull	Toe Rotation	Toe Circumduction
8	Place the inside base of each palm firmly below each anklebone. Move the hands rapidly back and forth (or up and down) in opposition to each other to effect a loose movement of the foot	Ankle Loosening	Hook in Ankles
9	Use both hands, side by side, with three or four fingers slide from toes to ankle area, then use the two middle fingers to circle around the ankles simultaneously three times. Finally, slide back to the toes	Effleurage	Dorsum and Ankle Stroking
10	Place thumbs on ball of foot. Put three or four fingers of each hand on the top/dorsum aspect of one foot, just below the toes. Crawl across the top of the foot horizontally so that the fingers meet in the middle. Open fingers so that hands lock; this avoids pinching the flesh	Chest and Abdominal Walk	
11	Use the 'heel' of the hand (Thenar eminence) to stroke down the inside of the foot following the curve of the spinal reflex	Inner Relaxer	Spine stroke
12	Grasp client's heel with a cupped left hand firmly holding the calcaneus between thenar and fingertips. Hold the upper dorsum of the same foot with the right hand keeping the foot at 90° to the leg. Exert a gentle but increasing pull towards practitioner's own chest and hold. To stretch ankle, knee and hip joints. Release pull slowly easing off. Repeat for other foot using opposite hands (useful for sciatica)	Heel Pull	Single Leg Stretch
13	Similar to 12 above but pulling both legs together. Cup each heel, one in each hand and grasping heel more with thenar to avoid thumb pressure into ankles. Gently pull legs toward chest and hold for 20 seconds then release slowly. To stretch and relieve pressure on hip, knee and ankle joints	Two Heel Pull	Double Leg Stretch
14	Place three fingers of each hand on dorsal chest reflex area of each foot. Place thumbs opposite on the plantar diaphragm line. Alternately push thumbs into diaphragm area and immediately pull fingers toward you and repeat with a smooth 'rocking', wave-like motion	Diaphragmatic Rocking	
15	Alternating pressure is applied to both solar plexus points with each thumb coinciding with the in and exhaling as the client takes up to 10 deep breaths*. Usually marks the end of a treatment	Solar plexus breathing	Deep breathing exercise

* Can make some clients light headed – not all may manage 10

However, should a practitioner wish to, or be requested to, provide an extra foot massage in addition to reflexology, this is a matter for the practitioner and client.

In situations such as pedal oedema and extreme stress an added foot or hand massage is very useful.

5.2 The Use of the Support Hand

The student must *understand* that at any one time whilst performing reflexology working techniques, one hand will be the *'working hand'* and the other will serve as the *'support or holding hand'*. The student should be able to *recall* that there are five distinct functions of the holding hand and be able to *describe* these as being:

- To support the foot being worked and to keep it stationary.
- To protect the foot from pressure to the opposite facet of the foot to where the pressure technique is directed, to avoid pinching and confusing the assessment of sensitive areas.
- To act as a platform off which the working hand fingers or thumb can lever.
- To spread or stretch an area of the foot so deep reflex points can be brought more to the surface to be accessed more easily by the working thumb or finger.
- To maintain client contact and transmit reassurance.

In addition to the above five functions, students should realise their own long-term health can be affected by incorrect technique and know how to employ the correct use of the holding hand to avoid repetitive strain injury to the joints of the working hand.

5.3 Reflexology Pressure Techniques

As explained above the various reflex points and areas have differences in nature: these reflex point types can be classified as:

A. *Large reflex areas* that may require a *moving technique*.
B. *Reflex points or small reflex areas* requiring a *precise, stationary technique*.
C. *Reflex points and areas* where a more investigative, *deeper technique* may be needed.
D. *Less accessible reflex points and other areas* requiring specific techniques.

Table of Techniques
Table 5B attempts to collate the existing variations as taught by different training organisations. This can be seen as an initial step to unification to make the task of regulation more effective. Some may view one technique as more valuable than another, or find that they can execute some more effectively due to existing experience or training.

As with relaxation techniques tutors should emphasise the need to assess the needs of the client in relation to pressure and vigour when delivering all reflexology pressure techniques. Students need to develop tactile and touch skills from the first day of training to be able to treat a wide range of clients who need adaptation of the techniques below to suit the needs of the client, from very light stroking touch to holding pressure depending on the stimulating, sedating or balancing effect required.

Table 5B

Type	Reflexology pressure techniques
A	*Large reflex areas that may require a moving technique:* 1. Forward moving alternating pressure or walking technique *('Thumb or Finger Walking')* 2. Stationary, 'bent thumb' technique – repeated over the entire reflex area 3. Index finger slide forward – return backward crawl (Example: Thoracic Lymphatics) 4. Index finger slide forward – pull distal joint back immediately, cover entire area and work back in reverse. (Example: Breast area)
B	*Reflex points and small reflex areas requiring a precise, stationary technique:* 1. Placing the thumb on a point and applying pressure *(Pin-pointing)* 2. Placing the thumb or index finger on a point and rotating *(Rotating)*
C	*Reflex points and areas where a more investigative, deeper technique may be needed:* 1. Placing the thumb on the reflex point, pushing in and bending the thumb as the wrist is dropped *('Hook in, Back up' Technique)* 2. Rocking the 'bent thumb' on the reflex point several times *(Rocking)* 3. Pinch between thumb and index finger with deep holding pressure, rotating both digits *(Pinch 'n' rotate)* (Example: Shoulder reflex – under little toe/finger)
D	*Less accessible reflex points and other areas requiring specific techniques:* 1. Reflex point and area requiring lateral edge of thumb walking (Example: Eyes and Ears, plantar ridge below toes) 2. Reflex point and area requiring index finger rolling technique (Example: Tops of toes – Brain, Top of Head) 3. Reflex points that can be worked by pin-pointing and rotating the foot into the index finger (Example: Ovaries/Testes, Uterus/Prostate) Thumb and Index finger pinch on webbing between toes (Example: Lymphatics)

Criteria for Techniques

Students should understand that any combination of the approved techniques in the table is appropriate, the criteria being:

- To *effectively treat* all reflex points and areas at a pressure sufficient *to detect a disordered reflex*
- To work all reflex points and areas *to achieve results safely* and never bringing *more than momentary discomfort* to the client.

Additions to the Table

The Reflexology Forum, as the emerging regulatory body, considers that Table 5B lists sufficient techniques to present standardised treatment to the discerning public. Any request for additional techniques may be considered by the Forum panel provided it is accompanied by an acceptable rationale.

5.4 Working Mediums

The student should ***understand*** that there may be a need to apply a working medium to the client's feet, or hands, in order to work without dragging, or slipping, when the texture of the skin not ideal. As there is still differing opinion and debate as to which medium is appropriate, the student should be able to ***analyse*** the advantages and disadvantages of the various recommended mediums and choose accordingly.

(This could be a subject for research as referred to in section 4.7. Students could demonstrate the ability to work at (academic) level 3 and (vocational) level 4 ***synthesise*** the appropriate conclusion to this debate and deliver the ideal medium.)

Examples of mediums
- Wherever possible, nothing at all
- *Liquid Talc**
- *Cornstarch**
- *Carrier Oil** – Essential Oils used by qualified practitioners only
- *Skin Lotion**
- *Skin Cream**
- Talcum powder** – During training consider clients with asthma/dust allergy – see Table 8B – adaptation

5.5 Positioning of Client and Practitioner

The student should be taught to understand that the positioning of client and practitioner is crucial to the effectiveness of a treatment, comfort and safety of the client and protection and well being of the practitioner.

5.5.1 Client position

Students should *know* how to set up the clinical area so that the client is positioned to receive an effective treatment whilst remaining in a secure and comfortable position for the entire session, which may last more than an hour. They should be able to *analyse* why the elements of correct positioning as listed here are important:

- The client's back and head are supported
- The back of the client's knees are supported
- The client's arms/hands are comfortably supported
- Wherever possible, the client should be in a semi-recumbent position that enables eye to eye contact with the practitioner
- The client's knees are slightly bent and supported
- The client's feet are supported:
    - At a height that permits safe and effective treatment

---

* The mediums in italics may allow the thumb and finger to slip and slide making it difficult for student beginners to identify minute reflex points.

** There have been concerns that talc is carcinogenic, yet unconfirmed. Some experienced practitioners still prefer this medium whilst taking care not to overuse and inhale.

– On a wide enough platform that permits all working and relaxation techniques to be performed on both feet at the same time

5.5.2 Practitioner position

Students should *know* how to set up the clinical area so that the practitioner is positioned to deliver an effective treatment whilst remaining in a comfortable position that does not compromise their well-being, for the entire session, which may last more than a hour. They should be able to *analyse* why the elements of correct positioning as listed here are important:

- The practitioner's back is supported
- The practitioner's chair is at the correct height
- Why the chair should or should not have castors
- Why all techniques are best delivered whilst remaining seated

5.6 Hand Reflexology

One of the aspects of the curriculum that would be more advantageous to visit *during a second year of the curriculum* is Hand Reflexology. This is similar in concept to reflexology to the foot, in that the hand and foot are referral areas and the reflex points and areas relate. However, there are also substantial differences that make it advisable to study this section once foot related treatment is well established.

5.6.1 Relaxation Techniques

The student will be required to *demonstrate* six hand reflexology relaxation techniques from Table 5C (overleaf).

5.6.2 Use of the support hand

The student should be able to *recall* the 5 functions of the support hand and *explain* why they are the same as for foot reflexology

5.6.3 Pressure Techniques

The student should be able to *describe* and *demonstrate* at least one pressure technique from each of A, B, C, D of Table 5B and adapt these to hand reflexology.

5.6.4 Working Mediums

The student should be able to *decide* which of the working mediums, if any, the client would like to be used on his hands and *demonstrate* working with this medium.

Table 5C: Hand Reflexology Relaxation Techniques

	Description	Name 1	Name 2
1	Gently place one palm on each dorsal surface of the hand with as much surface contact as possible. Hold for up to 30 seconds. Used to initiate client contact then go to number two:	Palming	'Greeting the hands'
2	Gently stroke from hand to forearm at the beginning of treatment, during the treatment and at the end	Effleurage	Stroking
3	With one palm on each palmar surface interlink fingers with client and perform several palmararflexions, sliding palms to perform alternate dorsiflexions, then evert and invert the hands several times, whilst using the holding hand to support the client's wrist. Used to ascertain mobility, detect resistance and encourage immediate relaxation. Use this prior to wrist rotation	Opening and Stretching Metacarpals	Dorsiflexion Palmarflexion Eversion Inversion
4	Support the metacarpals between thumb and fingers of one hand and support the heel of the wrist with the other. Rotate the hand and wrist slowly several times in each direction. Repeat for other hand.	Wrist Rotation	Circumduction
5	Stroke down the arm and slide off at the thumb, gently wringing as you go	Thumb Wringing	Thumb Pull
6	Gently wring and pull the fingers one at a time	Finger Wringing	Finger Pull
7	Alternating pressure is applied by the flat fist to the upper palmar area whilst other hand cradles the opposite dorsal aspect to spread the metacarpals. Repeat on other hand	Metacarpal Spread	Lung Press
8	Alternating pressure is applied with each thumb to both solar plexus points coinciding with the in and exhaling as the client takes up to 10 deep breaths*. Usually marks the end of a treatment	Solar Plexus Breathing	Deep Breathing Exercise

* Can make some clients light headed – not all may manage 10

5.6.5 Positioning of Client and Practitioner

The student must *know* how to set up the clinical area so that the client position meets the same needs as for the feet (see 5.5.1) and for Practitioner (see 5.5.2) Students must be made to realise that client personal space is invaded more during hand reflexology. Devices to put a barrier between client and practitioner such as pillow on lap, corner of a table, narrow desk, massage couch, podium or coffee table with cushions.

6 CLINICAL PRACTICE

> Recommended Teacher Contact Hours – **40**   Expected Home Study Hours – **80**

OVERVIEW OF THIS SECTION

The section Clinical Practice contains all the areas of skill and knowledge that the clinical reflexologist should be taught in order to deliver the techniques in section 5 to clients in a pleasant and safe manner and environment.

The section will therefore encompass the treatment itself, the practitioner him/herself, the practice environment and its management and the relationship to other practitioners and treatments, both conventional and within CAM.

The Treatment

The student should be led through all aspects of treatment. For ease of reference the presentation of this section 6 uses the format of the National Occupational Standards (NOS):

- Assessing the client's needs
  - Preparing to assess the client – **6.1**
  - Assessing the client – **6.2**
  - Agreeing action with the client – **6.3**
- Planning, providing and reviewing the reflexology programme
  - Planning the reflexology programme – **6.4**
  - Working the reflexes to promote healing – **6.5**
  - Enabling clients to treat themselves – **6.6**
  - Reviewing the effectiveness of the reflexology programme – **6.7**

Some of the following aspects of clinical practice are common to both of the above sections and their sub sections.

Many areas of the NOS classifications above have been covered in other course content sections of this curriculum (4 and 5; reflected in 7 & 8).

LEARNING OUTCOMES FOR SECTION 6

After completing this section of the curriculum the student will be able to:

6.1 *Demonstrate* how to **Prepare to Assess the Client**
Demonstrate the creation of a therapeutic environment in the classroom and *discuss* how to extend this to private practice

6.1.1   *Demonstrate* the preparation of a hygienic, calm, secure and private clinical area acceptable to all client groups *analysing* when to use music and aroma *Articulate* knowledge of hygiene terms and the characteristics of bacteria, viruses, fungi and common infestations, routes of transmission and the body's primary and secondary defences to infection and *state* how this knowledge informs hygiene practice

6.1.3   *State* the importance of preparing themselves physically, mentally and emotionally for treatment and *demonstrate* through *discussion* that their understanding of the terms 'spirituality' and 'grounding' is acceptable to all client groups and the profession

6.1.4   *Demonstrate* understanding and appreciation of Clinical Supervision and Continual Professional Development and an intention to make use of both provisions

6.2   *Demonstrate* how to **Assess the Client**

6.2.1   *Discuss* establishing a Therapeutic Relationship employing sensitivity and empathy, communication skill, professionalism and never abusing trust

6.2.2   *Demonstrate* the use of all senses, sight, hearing, smell and touch to initially assess the client

6.2.3   *Evaluate* and *demonstrate* the understanding and use of good consultation and communication skills, verbal and non-verbal, *recall* the four divisions of interpersonal space and the definition of counselling

6.2.4   *Demonstrate* awareness of confidentiality issues and how this relates to client records and handling of clients. *Demonstrate* knowledge of consent and continuous consent and how this relates to client records

6.2.5   *State* the definitions of Contraindication and Caution, *recall* which conditions and situations fall into these categories and *demonstrate* how to handle such a situation

6.2.6   *Define* the term 'diagnosis' and *discuss* to what extent reflexology relates to diagnosis and the practitioner's role in this

6.2.7   *Analyse* whether holism dictates that reflexology does not treat specific illness, whether reflexologists cure illness and whether reflexology can be used to control symptoms

6.3   *Demonstrate* Agreeing Action with the Client

6.3.1   *Evaluate* the importance of referral procedure, *state* the etiquette of contacting the client's doctor and *write* a professional letter, *state* situations when to refer to GP and continue with reflexology, when not to continue, when to refer straight to A & E, when to refer to another reflexologist or another CAM discipline

6.3.2   *Recall* the various Voluntary and Statutory Support Organisations that clients may fine useful and when and how to direct the client to them. *Articulate* how to help clients claim fees back from Private Health Care Plans

6.3.3   *Recall* a comprehensive list of other CAM disciplines; *define* what each discipline involves and if it is appropriate to use it alongside reflexology

6.4   *Demonstrate* Planning the Reflexology Programme

6.4.1   *Recall* the main tenets and general thrust of their own professional body's Code of Conduct and Ethics and *show* how these relate to reflexology practice

6.4.2   *Articulate* how to operate a small business and the issues relating to tax, accounts, and relevant legislation whether from home, from their own or at another's business premises. *Demonstrate* the production of a research, business and operational plan

6.4.3   *Evaluate* the need for appropriate insurance cover and *define* Public Liability; Professional Indemnity and Malpractice cover

6.5 *Demonstrate* **Working the Reflexes to Promote Healing** (see sections 4, 5, 7 and 8)

6.5.1 *Analyse* and *evaluate* the issues relating to the usual hour's length of a normal reflexology treatment, the duration of a number of treatments and the need for review, the idea and frequency of health maintenance treatments and when and how to discontinue treatment

6.5.2 *Articulate* how to adapt treatment to specific client types: Age Related – neonate, infant, under 16, elderly: Disability – mental, physical, wheelchair, without speech, hearing and vision: Cultural factors and diversity

6.5.3 *Demonstrate* understanding of the special issues relating to pregnant clients

6.5.4 *Analyse* and *evaluate* the special issues relating to supporting people with cancer

6.5.5 *Demonstrate* understanding of the need to follow a treatment pattern to miss nothing out of a treatment, keep to a time schedule, evaluate client progress and give reassurance to the client

6.6 *Demonstrate* **Enabling Clients to Treat Themselves**

6.6.1 *Analyse* the merits and disadvantages of giving self help advice and *state* when to do this, and how often and to what extent clients should treat themselves

6.6.2 *Analyse* the merits and disadvantages of the use of instruments in reflexology, why practitioners should never do this but how to advise clients on this subject

6.6.3 *Articulate* their understanding about prescribing that reflexology is the only thing a reflexologist can prescribe and that anything else, including water, is by opinion only

6.7 *Demonstrate* **Reviewing the Effectiveness of Reflexology**

6.7.1 *Demonstrate* how to record treatments effectively and consistently and when and why to review these at regular intervals – audit – in order to establish treatment effectiveness and *articulate* how to safely store records to ensure confidentiality

6.7.2 *Recall* common misunderstandings related to reflexology and *synthesise* how to reassure clients with the true facts

LEARNING OUTCOMES MAPPED AGAINST ASSESSMENT TOOLS
(See Appendix 2)

Tool	Learning Outcome Verbs
Case Studies	analyse; demonstrate; discuss; explain;
Client Studies	evaluate; list;
Home Treatments	evaluate; list; locate
Blank Feet/Hand Diagrams to locate Reflex Points/Areas	draw; locate; recall;
Blank Diagrams of Body Parts to Labels A&P Items	draw; locate; recall;
2000 to 5000-word Assignments At level 2 At level 3	analyse; assess; analyse; assess; critique, evaluate; synthesise;
Interim (Formative) Assessments (Written)	draw; locate; recall;
Interim (Formative) Assessments (Practical)	articulate, demonstrate; demonstrate understanding;
Final (Summative) Assessments (Written)	draw; locate; recall;
Final (Summative) Assessments (Practical)	demonstrate;
Professional Portfolio	analyse, articulate, list,
Interview	articulate, explain; list; recall; state;
Project: Research based or audit	analyse, design, evaluate, manage,

COURSE CONTENT SECTION 6

6.1 Creating a Therapeutic Environment

The student should know the importance of creating the correct setting for the treatment of clients, be able to analyse the reasons for pursuing courses of action and synthesise a therapeutic environment during classroom practical sessions (client studies) and outside the classroom (case studies).

6.1.1 Preparation of Clinical Environment

Students should know the importance of preparing the treatment area to be hygienic, calming, secure, private and acceptable to all clients.

Hygiene and Infection Control

Students' knowledge of Hygiene and Infection Control needs to extend to the ability to define the following terms: 'pathogenic' and 'micro organism'; the comparative definitions of 'sterilisation'; 'sanitation' and 'hygiene'. The difference between a *disinfectant* and an *antiseptic* must be known.

If students can relate the following facts of how the main groups of microorganisms operate to reflexology situations, best-practice of hygiene will naturally develop:

Bacteria

Knowledge of bacteria should extend to the classification of three types; coccus (round shape), bacillus (rod shaped) and spirillum (spiral shape), that they are not all pathogenic, the environmental conditions in which they thrive and the conditions that will destroy them or render their spores inert. Students should be able to identify the bacterial infections more likely to be encountered when practising reflexology such as: Staphylococcus – pus; Streptococcus – throat infections and TB.

Viruses

Knowledge of viruses should extend to the fact that they are always pathogenic and that, in their free and infectious form, cannot be considered to be living, as they do not grow, feed or respire. Thus, in the strictest sense, they cannot be 'killed'. Students should be able to identify the viral infections more likely to be encountered when practising reflexology such as: Verruca (plantar wart), the Common cold and Influenza.

Fungi

Knowledge of fungi should extend to the fact that, although they are related to plants, they lack chlorophyll and being unable to manufacture their own food have to live as parasites (obtaining food from living matter) or saprophytes (obtaining food from dead, organic matter). Knowledge should also extend to include they are not always pathogenic and the conditions in which they thrive: warm, moist and dark. Fungal infections often encountered by reflexologists should be known – Tinea Pedis (Athlete's Foot) and Candidiasis (Thrush).

Other infestations

Knowledge of other infestations can be limited to recognition and treatment of those likely to be encountered as contraindications in the UK (or the country where the course is being taught): e.g. Scabies, Head Lice and Fleas.

Routes of transmission of micro organisms and primary and secondary defences

Knowledge of the *routes* by which disease-causing micro-organisms can enter the body should extend to nose, mouth, eyes, ears, skin, and genito-urinary tract and an understanding of body fluid transmission. There should also be understanding of the primary (structural) and secondary (immune system) defences in place within the body to prevent this.

Integrating hygiene theory into practice

The student's knowledge of hygiene theory should inform their ability to employ best practice. Students should be able to describe and demonstrate best hygienic working practice in the clinical area extending to all hard surfaces* – walls, ceiling, doors and shelves, floor covering (hard and soft); furniture (hard and soft): equipment – treatment couch, chairs, stools, trolleys and any foot or nail care tools used**; the WC and any reception and waiting areas. Description and demonstration of best hygiene working practice should also extend to the client's feet (and hands); the practitioners' hands and hair and the hygiene procedure for any fabrics used – clothing and uniform, towels and couch and pillow covers.

6.1.2 Preparing a calm, secure, private and acceptable environment

Students must be aware of the importance of providing an environment that is fit for clinical practice but without the cold, emotionless qualities attributed to the term 'clinical': Students should be able to describe and evaluate the importance to the client of a calm, secure and private treatment area that will be acceptable to all types of client. They should be able to analyse why the structure, décor and furnishings of a clinic room may affect different clients and be able to reason on why a practitioner may choose not to personalise a room with religious or political decoration to the extent that it becomes unacceptable to certain clients.

Music, aromatic oils

Factors to consider; whether the practitioner would choose to play music or 'relaxing' sound recordings or use aromatherapy odours during a treatment will be covered in this section of a course. Students should be taught to weigh any assumed benefits of improved relaxation and a more pleasing environment with possible disadvantages. Verbal interaction with the client during a treatment can be invaluable to client assessment and music may signal that this is discouraged. Music is emotive and very personal and clients may not feel free to suggest the practitioner's choice is not their own. Both music and aromas can revive powerful negative memories as well as pleasant. Music can be turned off or changed instantly but an aroma that works for one client may be totally unsuitable for

---

*Awareness of reporting to the tutor unhygienic conditions in a college/school environment can be assessed

**Some training providers offer foot and nail care for reflexologists

the next, or for those within its reach, including the practitioner. Some 'pure' reflexologists have reasoned that music and aromatherapy are separate disciplines. Whatever the decision, the needs of the client transcend the wishes of the practitioner.

Assessment

Assessment of this part of the curriculum will usually have to be by written assignment or examination question as rarely would the student's own work in creating a clinical area be demonstrated for assessment. Practical assessment (client studies) will usually be on the school/college premises or clinical placement.

Risk assessment

Students should be able to demonstrate understanding of Risk Assessment procedure and documentation and be able to apply this to their own practice.

6.1.3 Preparation of Self, Practitioner

Knowledge of how practitioners can prepare themselves physically, mentally, emotionally and spiritually before treatment and developing strategies for maintaining personal protection during and after treatment should be covered in this part of the curriculum.

Spirituality

Discussion regarding the appropriate view of the term 'spiritual' must be included in this section. *Reflexology can benefit everyone and students must appreciate the importance of maintaining a neutral stance by using the term 'spiritual' in neither a religious nor mystical context.* Reflexology is compatible with conventional healthcare, and although an ancient art, this practice should be presented in the same light as any other medical science. As reflexology research is as yet at an early stage, care should be taken by training providers in using language that does not align reflexology with magic, fortune telling or astrology so as not to alienate conventional medical practitioners whose assistance in setting up clinical trials will be invaluable. It should be emphasised to students never to impose their personal beliefs, however sincerely held, upon a client.

Physical, mental and emotional preparation

Students should also consider the care and steps to be taken in preparing for clinical practice by taking care of themselves physically, with good nutrition, proper rest and life style. The good physical health of the practitioner will benefit the client. Consideration of how many clients it would be wise to treat in one day will benefit the student and devices that practitioners can use to prevent being emotionally drained should be discussed.

Grounding

The course should provide a balanced view of the importance of 'grounding', avoiding taking a too literal view. The practice of building into the treatment pattern a significant break between each client should be taught.

Assessment

As with 6.1 above, assessment of this part of the curriculum will usually have to be by written assignment or examination question as rarely could students demonstrate preparation of self.

6.1.4 Supervision, Clinical Supervisor

The course should include discussion and analysis of the subject of clinical supervision and the evaluation of paying for this service. Course tutors should be keen to see that clinical supervision has been set up so that following graduation new practitioners have a seamless transition to a support structure.

6.1.5 Continuing Professional Development (CPD)

As with clinical supervision, the course should include a consideration of Continuing Professional Development. Students can be given information that it can include a range of activities such as Literature review, attending Conferences and Workshops, enrolling on further Specialist Courses and Update days, Research Projects and Volunteer work.

6.2 Assessing the Client

The following aspects of 6.2 can be listed under the heading of assessing the client, although many will apply to all sections of clinical practice.

6.2.1 Establishing a Therapeutic Relationship

Students should be aware that a sensitive and empathetic manner should be adopted at all times. The practitioner should develop excellent communication and client handling skills. These are necessary in building a rapport with the client and ensuring that maximum information is elicited in order to assess the client's requirements and plan a suitable treatment. Professionalism should be demonstrated at all times and the trust between the client and the therapist should never be abused.

6.2.2 Using all senses to initially assess the client

Students should be taught to use all their senses to initially assess the client. They should consider that this process starts before the consultation and an experienced practitioner will begin assessment from the first point of contact, which could be as soon as they first *see* their client. Initial assessment could even be said to be by *hearing* when making the appointment, by telephone. A device covering this could be to compile a list of as many aspects of assessment as possible for each sense – before during and after treatment. Such a list could include:

Sight

Posture and gait, body language, demeanour, facial expression, care and type of attire and grooming, facial expression, pallor, eyes ('windows to the soul'). Foot disorders, which can *cause* problems, callus, heloma and ingrowing nails – (e.g. ingrown nail is often associated with headache) and foot disorders, which can *signify* problems (e.g. heloma [corn] may be a sign of a posture/gait problem). Uneven wear to shoes.

Hearing
Voice – pitch, pace, power; sharp intake of breath; silence; breathing – pitch, pace, power.

Smell
Natural body odour as well as smells due to poor personal hygiene, breath, smoking, and heavy perfume.

Touch
(The 'Ts'): Temperature, tension, tone, texture, tenderness, tremors, and ticklishness. Though covered in section 5, the importance of touch in the assessment of the client's feet (and hands) before, during and after the treatment cannot be overemphasised.

6.2.3 Consultation and Communication Skills

Some have used the expression 'counselling' in connection with reflexology training and whilst undoubtedly the skills that clinical reflexologists need are similar, counselling can be two-year (diploma) or three-year (degree level) training. The term to be employed to cover the needed training will be consultation and/or communication skills. Students need to be trained in these skills to assess the client's needs adequately *but should not be led to believe they will be qualified in counselling upon completion of this curriculum.*

Definition of communication
The definition of communication should be recalled by the reflexology student as 'the transmitting and receiving of information'.

Verbal skills
The following aspects of verbal communication should be taught and there should be discussion on how they may applied to reflexology: Active listening (which is in fact non-verbal in the sense that it is silence); types of questions – open, closed, leading and probing; types of responses – reflective, restating, clarifying and summarising.

Non-verbal skills
The following aspects of non-verbal communication should be taught and there should be discussion on how they may be applied to reflexology and in particular the 'reflexology package':

Proximity/personal space (see interpersonal distance); orientation and posture; gestures – body and facial; eye contact/gaze; hand contact/touch; privacy and paralanguage.

Interpersonal distance
The definitions and divisions of interpersonal distance are relevant to reflexology:

- Intimate Space: 0–18" – Lovers and intimate family
- Personal Space: 18"–4' – Friends

- Social Space: 4'–12' – Business & casual acquaintances
- Public Space: 12'–25' – Formal interactions

(Hall, E 1983)

That the practitioner is able to touch the client's feet without invading their personal space is significant in reflexology and does explain why some are less comfortable with hand reflexology.

Definition of counselling

The definition of counselling should be recalled by the reflexology student as: 'A process where a person in an understanding atmosphere enables another by purposeful conversation to make his own decisions given the choices available to him'.

Counselling skills

The aspects of counselling skills to be considered during this reflexology practitioner training should be: Difference between listening and hearing; levels of listening; physical and psychological barriers to effective listening; confidentiality; knowing practitioner limitations and when to refer.

6.2.4 Confidentiality

The issue of confidentiality applies to all aspects of reflexology such as communication and counselling and treatment recording and students should be aware of the following principles:

All conversations within a treatment are confidential and must not be repeated outside the client/practitioner situation.

Some clinics have a policy of sharing information regarding clients, but this should be confirmed with the client and permission given beforehand.

If students are working on each other in class confidentiality also applies.

Case and client studies

Where written records are used in portfolios all sensitive information and personal details should be removed. Clients can be identified and indexed by colours and/or numbers and the student can keep a secure master/key file away from the portfolio.

Data Protection

Students should be reminded to check that their process for recording written and electronic information conforms to the Data Protection Act.

Client Consent

All students should be able to write about and demonstrate that before commencing the treatment and after completing the consultation form the client should sign it, agreeing that the information given to the practitioner is correct. This will imply they are willing to go ahead with the treatment. It would complete the contract and reassure the client if the practitioner countersigns this to agree that the information will be treated in strict confidence. The fact that some reflexologists still do not obtain a signature or even keep records of treatments does not mean students should not be trained to do this. Insurance may be invalid and there could be legal implications if practitioners cannot demonstrate the organised keeping of records and establish consent.

Continuous Consent

Provision should be made for change of circumstances. For example, if a client became pregnant, after having written 'no' to the question 'is there any chance you may be pregnant' the record will no longer be accurate and the situation should be reviewed and ongoing consent agreed. A simple endorsement can be added to the treatment record and signed and dated by both client and practitioner.

Clients should be aware that their consent might be withdrawn at any time before a new treatment session commences.

6.2.5 Contraindications and Cautions

See Appendix 3.

The issue of what constitutes a contraindication to reflexology led to an extensive task in the preparation of this curriculum. Almost every major reflexology text had a different list of contraindications ranging from none to 'any condition that may be affected by the treatment'. (See introduction to Appendix 3.)

A task force was set up as part of the Education and Training group to consider this issue and this panel of experts extensively examined the rationale for each of the suggested contraindications.

The resulting list was decided to include what should be kept as contraindications (where treatment should not take place at all) and cautions (where treatment could continue with caution or with adaptation). All items on the list can be considered a valid teaching point for discussion and analysis with students.

6.2.6 Diagnosis

Students should be taught that it is not their prerogative to offer a conventional medical diagnosis to their client or furnish an allopathic label to their condition. A doctor often has to use other members of the healthcare team before he can decide upon an accurate diagnosis and sometimes clients expect reflexologists to do the same in a single treatment. It is true that sometimes the client's feet (and hands) can be 'devastatingly accurate in giving an instant picture of a person's health condition' (Kunz & Kunz 1984) and a trained practitioner can at times contribute vital information which can initiate, further inform, confirm or clarify a doctor's diagnosis. However, the above source warns that reflexology can also be misinterpreted totally. This emphasises the need for this extended core curriculum and its rigorous assessment.

6.2.7 Treatment of specific illness

Students should be helped to analyse whether the concept of holism dictates that reflexology does not treat specific illness. Whilst a practitioner would never promise a cure, clients present with specific illness and their initial focus is on that. The student can weigh the fact that the treatment pattern will normally treat the entire person but with emphasis to the areas that the practitioner decides during the assessment of the client

(Section 8). If reflexology does not treat specific illness at all then most research projects currently underway would be flawed in that they usually attempt to measure the effectiveness of reflexology treatment in relation to a very specific aspect of ill health.

6.3 Agreeing action with the client

6.3.1 Referral

Students should be aware of the importance of using correct referral procedure when accepting referrals from other practitioners within and outside the health service and when and how to go about suggesting clients visit another practitioner as well as, or instead of, continuing to treat them personally.

Etiquette of referral

The etiquette of contacting the client's doctor, for example, should be taught during the course and letter writing practised. The balance between showing due respect and being subservient should be analysed and the correct procedure for contacting the GP or client's consultant should be discussed.

To client's GP and continue treatment

Situations where clients should be advised to visit their doctor should be discussed with students. These could include occasions where the reflexology treatment and client's information makes the practitioner suspect that further investigations and/or conventional treatment may be advisable but would not expect to lead to a contraindication. For example, a known diabetic who may need his medication dosage changing but who has been having reflexology for a period of time could still continue with treatment.

To client's GP and not continue treatment

These could include occasions where the reflexology treatment and client's information makes the practitioner suspect further investigations and/or conventional treatment may be advisable but may lead to a contraindication. These situations may include a suspected contagious infection or lead to a test where improving the situation by reflexology treatment may mask a doctor's test. This could be an undiagnosed diabetic condition.

To A & E immediately

Students should discuss emergency situations that may arise and require quick action. A reflexologist may be the first to recognise gangrene, a client may collapse, suffer a CVA (stroke), have their first fit (or one that lasts longer than 5 minutes) or haemorrhage.

To another practitioner

Another reflexologist

The discussions should extend to situations that may require the client to transfer to another reflexology practitioner which could include personality clash, the client requesting a different gender, the practitioner feeling inadequate or recognising their limitations.

Another discipline

Referral discussion should also extend to other CAM or conventional disciplines that may be suitable instead of or in addition to reflexology. These disciplines are listed in **6.3.3** but this referral section requires the student to be able to recognise the type of conditions that would be suited to which other disciplines. For example, *mechanical* or *structural problems* would be better suited to *manipulative* treatments such as Osteopathy, Chiropractic, Alexander Technique or Physiotherapy whereas *systemic* conditions like *eczema* would be better suited to Homeopathy, TCM or Herbal treatment. Students should be able to recall the list **6.3.3.**

6.3.2 Support Services: Voluntary and Statutory Organisations

Students should appreciate that voluntary and statutory support services may have a role in managing a client's condition and it may help the client if the practitioner was informed to suggest such a service where appropriate.

Voluntary

Student should know the area of focus, the range of services, type of support and advice offered by voluntary support services, limited to: Cruse, WRVS, Age Concern, Help the Aged, RNIB, RNID, CAB, Samaritans, RELATE, AA, and AIDS Helpline.

Statutory

Similarly, in the case of statutory services, being limited to: Social Services, the Benefits Agency, Local Borough Housing Departments, Medical or Health Centres and NHS Advice Line/Alert.

Private Health Care Plans

It may help some clients to sustain reflexology treatments if their care plan included reflexology. Commercial implications make it the responsibility of the practitioner to find out which plans include reflexology as a reclaimable expense and pass this information to their clients.

6.3.3 Relationship to other complementary therapies

Students should be able to recall the minimum list of other CAM disciplines below and be aware of the followings facts for each:

* What does it involve?
* What type of treatment is it? Systemic; manipulative; etc
* Can one receive it alongside reflexology?

List of CAM disciplines:

Acupuncture, Alexander Technique, Aromatherapy, Bach Flower Remedies, Bowen Technique, Chiropractic, Healing – spiritual and natural, Herbalism, Homeopathy, Hypnotherapy, Iridology, Kinesiology, Neurolinguistic Programming (NLP), Osteopathy, Physiotherapy, Reiki, Remedial and Therapeutic Massage, Therapeutic Touch, Shiatsu, Traditional Chinese Medicine, Yoga.

6.4 Planning, providing and reviewing the reflexology programme:

6.4.1 Code of Practice and Ethics

Students will not be expected to recall whichever Reflexology organisation's Code of Practice and Ethics their school/college/awarding body uses, but only know the main tenets and state their general thrust and how they apply to reflexology practice. In addition, they should be able to explain the reason or rationale for the inclusion in the Code of each tenet. Students should be able to state valid and relative examples of how the stipulations of the Code are implemented in Reflexology practice.

6.4.2 The Clinic – Practice and Business management

Students must be aware of the fundamental principles under which a small business operates. As this could extend to a two-year practitioner curriculum it is expected that the student will have plans to establish their own business or work in a clinical healthcare environment. In either situation the understanding of the basic principles of the following areas of business will be invaluable:

- Business models for practitioners and their relative merits limited to:
  - self-employment at home, in a clinic or a mobile service,
  - an employed position within a clinic/salon
  - business, sole proprietor
  - business, employing staff
  - voluntary model, e.g. hospice
- Income Tax/National Insurance Requirements for the Self-employed
- Methods of Book Keeping and keeping financial records
- Legal constraints on therapists including the Trade Descriptions Act, HASAWA, Licensing and Prohibited Appellation Legislation. Recall of legal statements or legislation will not be required other than those of the Prohibited Appellation and Trade Descriptions Act (see Appendix 5: Current Legislation of which students should be aware).

Students should be able to produce:

- Research Plan:
  - Catchment area
  - List of competitors
  - Details and charges of other practitioners in area
- Business Plan
  - Set up Costs
  - Overheads
  - Cash Flow Forecast
- Operational Plan
  - Advertising and Marketing designs, cards, leaflets
  - Design and Layout of clinical area
  - Equipment list
  - Risk Assessment
  - Treatment records, plans for security of these

6.4.3 Insurance

Students should discuss, analyse and evaluate the need for insurance to cover their professional and business activities. Student insurance should be able to be in place should they request or need it. They should be aware to investigate whether the insurance they eventually obtain covers treatment of clients with any medical condition without written permission from the GP.

Professional Indemnity

Students will be expected to know that professional indemnity is to cover the delivering of clinical reflexology treatment.

Public Liability

Students will be expected to know that public liability is to cover all risks in relation to working with clients and the operation of a business dealing with members of the public.

6.5 Working the reflexes to promote healing

6.5.1 Treatment

Length

Students should be taught that for the Core Curriculum which relates to 'Classical', 'Standard' or 'Pure' Reflexology (as opposed to specialised, developed types of treatment as would be learned usually via CPD) the length of a treatment is normally 45 minutes to 1 hour. Treatment should meet the client's needs at the time. For example see **6.5.2**.

Duration

Students should know to consider the client's needs with this. Treatments would normally be reviewed to give the client and/or practitioner the option to suspend treatment after four/six sessions if there are no *reactions* (good or unpleasant) and discontinue treatment after ten sessions if there is no *benefit* at all experienced by the client or detected by the practitioner.

Maintenance

Students should know this would vary according to the client's needs. After initial treatment the client may only require one session per week, month or quarter or be seasonal and will vary between clients and conditions presenting will depend on ongoing consent and treatment reviews.

Discontinuing

The client and the practitioner must feel free to discontinue the treatment plan at any point. The reason for discontinuing the treatment should be ascertained and discussed if appropriate. The options to suspend on the basis of no reaction and discontinue if no benefit not only protect the client from exploitation but also free the practitioner.

6.5.2 Treatment Adaptation

Every clinical treatment involves adaptation to the client. However, students should consider the following range of specific client types to integrate theory into practice. Assessment should cover as wide a range as possible. In all cases ensure that the treatment has been fully explained and understood.

Age

Neonate

Very short treatment length and maybe gentle, light pressure – the foot could be smaller than the practitioner's thumb.

Infant

With both infant and neonate the emphasis will be on showing the parents how to deliver the treatment themselves. Parents will sign consent on treatment record. Give a short, 15-minute maximum treatment, usually with light pressure.

Children under 16

Students should know to obtain parent's written permission. Light pressure only is usually needed depending on the stature of the child. Keep explanations simple but do not underestimate the child's intelligence. Ensure extra reassurance, as a child may be shy or self-conscious. Home self-help advice should be explained to the child but also confirmed to the parent. Issues and legalities of always having parent/guardian present, suspected abuse and relative confidentiality must be explored. *Students must be alert to make sure the parents/guardians are not withholding needed medical treatment from their child as a practitioner could be implicated if reflexology treatment was given at the time.*

Young female

Students should be aware of possible additional issues (pregnancy, menstrual difficulties, eating disorders etc). Ensure extra reassurance if necessary and be extremely professional.

Elderly

Client may be hard of hearing, have poor vision or be less mobile. Take extra time to explain treatment and ensure client understands each time. Reassurance. Use a shorter treatment and/or less pressure if necessary – elderly clients may have less adipose tissue, brittle bones, crêpe-like skin and may be arthritic. Ensure firm support for this client and extra assistance on and off the treatment couch/chair. Ensure client understands any aftercare advice, write this down or give information to the carer.

Disability

Students must know how to use appropriate pressure and adapt technique if necessary. Maintain client dignity at all times. Carer may need to be present during treatment. Adaptation to the client position may be necessary during treatment.

Mental

In addition to the above be very reassuring. Ensure that any explanations are given to a carer or parent if appropriate. Take safety precautions if instability is an issue, such as using a chaperone, ensuring a clear escape route and making sure others know where you are. Some situations may be contraindicated. Special training, possibly via CPD may be advantageous.

Physical
If client cannot weight bear then do not lift unless you are qualified to do so. Technique may need considerable adaptation.

Wheelchair
If client cannot weight bear then do not lift unless you are qualified to do so. Ensure that the brakes are on before commencing treatment. When supporting client's legs ensure the knees are supported too. Practitioners' own health and safety are important when using adapted technique. If the client suffers from leg muscle spasms adapt to these and avoid cold wipes.

Without speech
The client's interpreter may be required to remain in the room during the treatment – always address the client NOT the interpreter. Write down any information or establish a method of communication before commencing the treatment.

Physically hard of hearing
Similar to above. Ensure a place for guide dog if necessary.

Visually impaired
Be especially observant and attentive as client gets on and off of the plinth or chair. Ensure are no areas where this client could trip or collide. Remember to explain what your intentions are before starting the treatment. Ensure a place for guide dog if necessary. Ensure you give full explanations and possibly copies to take away of any written documentation and describe the foot charts. Explore issue of the blind and written consent.

Cultural Factors
Students should in all cases use appropriate pressure and adapt their hold or position if necessary. The must be able to state how they can maintain client dignity at all times. Students should be aware of different cultural customs and needs such as a same gender practitioner, not exposing too much area of skin. They must respect all cultures.

Diversity
Students should acknowledge diversity in all situations and give due respect.

*The following two sections **6.5.3** Pregnancy and **6.5.4** Cancer Care have been given special consideration, as both require hours to be allocated to them on the course and are both recommended to be subjects for CPD.*

6.5.3 Pregnancy

Students should be aware that two lives are involved. Pregnancy would be a useful post-graduate training subject, because of its special nature and its history of being commonly presented as a contraindication.

However, during the body of the course, the Reflexology Forum recommendation is that 20 hours (6 teacher contact) are dedicated to this subject, ideally delivered by a midwife also qualified in reflexology where this is possible, or accompanied/replaced by a suitably qualified and experienced practitioner and that the following aspects are covered:

- The complete process of pregnancy from conception to delivery
- Common complications of pregnancy and methods of treatment
- Termination/miscarriage – physiological & psychological changes
- Methods and interventions of delivery – likely outcomes on mother
- Common infertility problems and the medical treatments available
- Awareness of any legal responsibilities
- How to adapt reflexology treatment to accommodate mother's needs

6.5.4 Cancer Care

Although cancer has previously been classed as a contraindication, reflexology is increasingly being used to support people with cancer. The nature of the treatment, including the various aspects of the 'reflexology package', make it an ideal complementary therapy to use at any stage or involvement in the cancer journey. However, treating cancer patients requires a specific knowledge and experience to work with confidence in the specialist area of supportive and palliative care. It is important that CPD courses are undertaken before working with vulnerable cancer patients.

The allocation of 20 hours (6 teacher contact) of the practitioner course needs to be related to cancer care, ideally delivered by a practitioner and qualified teacher who specialises in using reflexology with people with cancer.

Following this allocation, students should be able to:

- *understand* the nature of the disease, cancer and its progression
- *be aware of* and *implement* the published National Guidelines for Supportive and Palliative Care
- *know* the common types of cancer
- be able to *define* the term oncology
- *be familiar with* the main treatments for cancer and how they are applied – chemotherapy; radiotherapy, surgery
- *know* the side effects of cancer treatments and be *aware* of how protracted treatment impacts upon patient's and carer's lives
- be able to *adapt* reflexology to cancer treatment side effects – nausea, fatigue, oedema, pain, constipation, neutropenia, neuropathy
- *relate to* the emotional impact of diagnosis and body image upon the patient and family
- *develop strategies* to handle the emotional impact from working with people with cancer and *plan* for clinical supervision
- *analyse* contraindications and when to use caution
- *dispel* myths related to reflexology stimulating cancer growth and spread and practitioner contamination from chemotherapy and radiation.

- *provide* a complete, 1 hour treatment for maximum benefit
- *articulate* the importance of developing a patient and carer treatment package that will put bereavement treatment help in place before death

6.5.5 Treatment Pattern

A number of treatment patterns exist. The original approach to treatment was to treat first the Right Foot and then the Left Foot. However, some may now follow a sequence where the Left Foot is treated first, then the Right or include treatment to the body in sequence involving both feet together. All methods have their merits. Some authorities reason that many reflex points or areas are reflected on both feet and working these as a unit rather than in isolation is more effective. The colon, urinary (renal) system and solar plexus are examples of such areas.

The pattern will be dependent on the training school method being taught. Students should be encouraged to analyse all approaches to treatment pattern and critically examine rationale when given.

All treatment patterns or sequences will involve treatment to ALL reflex points and areas of the feet. See **4.6.2** and **4.8.**

6.6 Enabling Clients to Help Themselves

6.6.1 Self Help

Methods

Students should be able to weigh the advantages against the disadvantages of giving advice about self help to the client, and come to the conclusion that some clients may benefit from the self-working, or treatment by a partner or family member. Not all clients will want to do this, some will benefit greatly. Students should be aware to monitor this each treatment.

Frequency and extent

All students should know to advise clients that they will benefit from only using two to four reflex points or areas. More than this will be impracticable. Clients should routinely spend up to fifteen minutes daily on self help most will not sustain longer. There are occasions when 'first aid' self help is valuable and students should be aware of examples where they could suggest this, such as working the Thumb (or great toe) for headache, the adrenals for allergic reactions (Kunz and Kunz, page 69) or the Solar Plexus (Coeliac Ganglion) for stress.

6.6.2 Use of Instruments

By the practitioner

There is a plethora of instruments and mechanical devices on sale in shops and on the Internet purporting to deliver 'reflexology' treatment. Students should be helped to evaluate the practice used by some therapists of using instruments to access reflex points and areas during reflexology treatment. Factors such as the danger of damaging the client's feet (and hands) by lack of pressure control, the danger of cross infection, the lack of professionalism using gimmicky devices, the absence of therapeutic, reassuring touch and the inability to detect the nature of the reflexes by touch should be able to be recalled by students in examination and help them reject the idea of using anything but their hands and fingers for treating clients.

By clients themselves

However, some of the above factors do not apply to clients using an instrument upon themselves and cannot be used to deter their use in self-help. Students should know not to recommend the use of tools; implements and self help instruments by clients as the circumstances of use are beyond the practitioner's control. If a client has been given or bought such a device students should be aware to advise against the dangers of damage, infection, desensitisation or hypersensitivity and overuse.

Use of instruments could never replace treatment by a practitioner.

6.6.3 Prescribing

Reflexology students should know that the only thing they are to be qualified to prescribe is reflexology, in that they prescribe a treatment after the initial consultation and the decision to continue. Self-help can also be prescribed. Anything else is outside the boundaries of reflexology and the temptation to prescribe should be curtailed. Even the routine instruction to drink more water would be prescribing if an amount were mentioned. Suggestion and opinion is the only option. Even if the practitioner is additionally qualified to permit prescription students should be taught to analyse whether treatments should be mixed in the same session and whether they should 'wear one hat at a time'.

6.7 Reviewing the effectiveness of the reflexology programme

6.7.1 Treatment Recording

All relevant information regarding the client should be recorded accurately and legibly, ensuring confidentiality at all times. Treatment records should be kept in a secure locked cabinet only available to be read by the practitioner and client who have signed the record. If a client transfers to another practitioner it would be preferable for them to take their original records with them leaving a transfer note in their place. As reflexology becomes established the need for a universal recording system increases so that clients' treatment records can be effectively referred to when transferred to another practitioner.

Audit

To objectively review the effectiveness of their treatment students should be encouraged to plan to audit their practice at regular intervals. Following the six (four) and ten guidelines referred to in **6.5.1** individual clients should be monitored for effectiveness and continued treatment.

6.7.2 Common misunderstandings

Part of the course should be a consideration of the many myths and common misunderstandings that have evolved around the theory and practice of reflexology. The higher level nature of this course will help students appreciate the value of respectfully challenging the 'rules' some of which are in place historically without any rationale whilst others exist based on best practice and years of practitioner experience.

The Contraindication and Caution list (section A3.6 in Appendix 3) is an example of challenging and examining rationale.

Examples of such common misunderstandings to be examined by students could be:

'Reflexology can precipitate ...:
* *A heart attack*
* *An epileptic seizure*
* *A miscarriage*
* *A hypoglycaemic attack*
* *The spread of cancer cells to secondary sites'*

7 ANATOMY AND PHYSIOLOGY

> Recommended Teacher Contact Hours – **50**   Expected Home Study Hours – **150**

INTRODUCTION

In accordance with the holistic nature of reflexology as complementary medicine, the eleven distinct systems of the human body should be studied from the viewpoint that they work synergistically, and as a complete, integrated organism.

The statement above becomes more relevant if a training programme includes the delivery of A & P as a module separate from reflexology.

Either the A & P instructor or the reflexology teacher, ideally both, must include teaching techniques for relating biological information to reflexology. A question such as 'In what ways can receiving reflexology treatment affect the .... system' will direct the student to commence integrating A&P into reflexology.

The curriculum also must contain an overview of the human body including basic histology and awareness of anatomical terms.

Learning outcomes for the minimum year are written in plain type and the items **in bold type** may be **visited later** in that period **or during a second year** if the training provider structures a longer or two year programme.

Students are to achieve both sets of learning outcomes to be a reflexologist and attain practitioner status.

LEARNING OUTCOMES FOR SECTION 7

By the end of the course the student should be able to:

7.1	*Recall* the eleven body systems
7.2	*Define* terms cell, tissue and organ
7.2.2	*Name* the types of cell and tissue. ***Describe* more detailed cell structure/ function/division.**
7.2.3	*Define* homeostasis **and homeodynamics, negative and positive feedback, *cite* an example of each.** *Understand* the effect of Lifestyle and Stress upon health.
7.2.4	*Demonstrate* the anatomical position, *understand* its importance to reflexology theory and be able *to label* the terms in Table 7.4 on a blank diagram
7.3	*Recall* the component parts of the integumentary system, *locate* these on a blank diagram and *define* the word 'integument'
7.3.1	*Describe* the structure and function of the skin, ***describe* how disorders are evidenced in skin**
7.3.2	*Describe* the structure and function of hair
7.3.3	*Describe* the structure and function of the nails
7.4	*Recall* the component parts of the respiratory system, *locate* these on a blank diagram and *state* the five stages of respiration
7.4.1	*Describe* the structure of the respiratory system

7.4.2   *Describe* the function of the respiratory system including the composition of air and the mechanism of respiration. ***Describe*** in *detail* **the effect smoking has upon respiration**

7.5   *Recall* the component parts of the Cardiovascular system and *locate* these on a blank diagram

7.5.1   *Describe* the structure and function of the heart and of the pulmonary circulatory system

7.5.2   *Describe* the structure and function of the blood

7.5.3   *Describe* the difference between the structure and function of the arteries, veins and capillaries. ***Describe*** in *detail* **the connection between the spleen, the liver and the blood**

State the factors affecting blood pressure. **Understand how blood pressure is measured and controlled by the body,** *demonstrate* **how to measure it by means of a sphygmomanometer**

7.6   *Recall* the component parts of the Lymphatic system, *locate* these on a blank diagram and *state* its basic structure as being a subsidiary circulatory system *describing* its primary functions.

7.6.1   *Describe* the structure and functions of lymph fluid.

Describe the structure and functions of lymph vessels, with specific details of the thoracic and lymphatic ducts

Describe the structure and functions of lymph nodes and nodules, with specific details of the spleen and thymus.

7.6.2   ***Describe*** **the action of the autoimmune system and how to recognise infection**

7.7   *Recall* the component parts of the Digestive system and *locate* these on a blank diagram

7.7.1   *Describe* the location and structure of the alimentary canal from the mouth through to the anus

Describe the function of the alimentary canal and all its parts

7.7.2   *Describe* the structure and functions of the accessory organs, liver, gall bladder and pancreas

7.7.3   *Recall* the timings of the different stages of digestion as food passes down the alimentary canal

7.7.4   ***Demonstrate*** **knowledge of food chemistry** *labelling* **enzymes and digestion stages on chart**

7.7.5   *Demonstrate* knowledge of basic nutrition and how balanced diet aids health, *recall* knowledge of vitamins and minerals and *demonstrate* a balanced view of dietary advice and water intake

7.8   *Recall* the component parts of the Urinary (renal) system and *locate* these on a blank diagram

7.8.1   *Describe* the location and structure of the kidneys and ureters; bladder and urethra

7.8.2   *Describe* the composition of urine, fluid balance and **the mechanism by which the kidneys affect blood pressure**

7.9   *Recall* the component parts of the Endocrine system, *locate* these on a blank diagram and *define* the terms endocrine and hormone

Describe the structure and functions of the pituitary gland and the hypothalamus and *recall* the names, targets and actions of the pituitary hormones by completing an unfinished table

7.9.1   *Describe* the structure and functions of the pineal gland

7.9.2   *Describe* the structure and functions of the thyroid gland

7.9.3   *Describe* the structure and functions of the parathyroid glands

7.9.4   *Describe* the structure and endocrine functions of the thymus

7.9.5   *Describe* the structure of the adrenal glands, the hormones and functions of the adrenal cortex and adrenal medulla

7.9.6   *Describe* the structure and endocrine functions of the Islets of Langerhans of the pancreas

7.9.7   *Describe* the endocrine functions of the male and female gonads
Recall the other locations in the body where hormones are produced and their effects

7.10   *Recall* the component parts of both the male and female Reproductive systems and *locate* these on a blank diagram

7.10.1   *Describe* the structure and functions of female reproductive organs, internal, external and breasts

7.10.2   *Describe* the structure and functions of the male reproductive organs and sperm

7.10.3   *Describe* the process of conception from the production of gametes to the birth process.

7.10.4   *Describe* the process of menstruation and the hormones involved

7.10.5   *Demonstrate knowledge* of infertility, its causes, the options available for assisted conception **and the how reflexology can aid this**

7.10.6   *Describe* the processes that happen to the bay's heart, pulmonary and hepatic blood vessels at birth and how 'hole in the heart' occurs

7.11   Recall the component parts of the nervous system and locate these on a blank diagram

7.11.1   *Describe* the structure and functions of the central nervous system, the areas of the brain, the spine and cerebrospinal fluid

7.11.2   *Describe* the structure and functions of the peripheral nervous system, *identifying* cranial, spinal, afferent and efferent nerves

7.11.3   *Describe* the structure and functions of the autonomic nervous system, *recall* the effects of the sympathetic and parasympathetic systems and *describe* the anomaly of the solar plexus

7.11.4   *Describe* the main types of neurones, components of nerve cells and *restate* their function

7.11.5   *Describe* the structure and functions of the organs of special sense; the skin, tongue, nose, eye and ear. ***Describe* in detail the main receptors in the skin and *locate* these on a diagram**

7.12   *Recall* the component parts of the Skeletal system and *know* its principal functions

7.12.1   *Recall* the number of bones in the body, *label* a blank skeletal diagram with the bones from Table 14.3 and label blank foot and hand skeletal diagrams in their entirety

7.12.2   *Understand* the function of bone marrow and its role in the production of blood cells

7.12.3   *Understand* the tissue structure and suitability of cartilage and the structure and function of ligaments

7.12.4   *Know* the structure and composition of bone and *understand* the terms for bone shape

7.12.5   *Complete* Table 7.12.5 for the classification of joint types giving examples of each

7.13   *Recall* the component parts of the Muscular system and *know* its principal function

7.13.1   *Recall* the number of muscles in the body, the three main types of muscle, *know* the terms relating to the characteristics of muscle and recognise the sites of muscle insertion and origin on the actual leg, foot, arm and hand

7.13.2   *Understand* what type of tissue comprise tendons and how their function differs from ligaments

LEARNING OUTCOMES MAPPED AGAINST ASSESSMENT TOOLS
(See Appendix 2)

Tool	Learning Outcome Verbs
Case Studies	analyse; cite, demonstrate; describe, discuss; explain
Client Studies	describe, evaluate, list
Home Treatments	describe, evaluate, list; locate
Blank Feet/Hand Diagrams to locate Reflex Points/Areas	draw locate, recall
Blank Diagrams of Body Parts to Labels A&P Items	describe, draw; label, locate, recall
2000 to 5000-word Assignments	
At level 2	analyse, assess, cite, demonstrate understanding & knowledge, describe, state
At level 3	analyse, assess; cite, critique, describe, evaluate; synthesise
Interim (Formative) Assessments (Written)	cite, describe, draw; locate; recall
Interim (Formative) Assessments (Practical)	articulate, cite, demonstrate; demonstrate understanding & knowledge, describe
Final (Summative) Assessments (Written)	cite, demonstrate understanding describe, draw; locate; recall
Final (Summative) Assessments (Practical)	cite, demonstrate, demonstrate understanding & knowledge, describe
Professional Portfolio	analyse, articulate, cite, describe, list
Interview	articulate, cite, demonstrate understanding & knowledge, describe, explain; list; recall; state
Project: Research based or audit	analyse, critique, describe, design, manage, evaluate, state, synthesise

COURSE CONTENT FOR SECTION 7

7.1 Overview of Body systems

Students should know the eleven body systems to be:

- Integumentary
- Respiratory
- Cardiovascular
- Lymphatic
- Digestive
- Urinary (renal)
- Endocrine
- Reproductive
- Nervous
- Skeletal
- Muscular

Commonly Encountered Diseases and Disorders

As each body system is studied there should be a consideration of the related common diseases and disorders integrating with **Table 7.2** and **Section 8**.

Health professionals

Students who embark upon a reflexology course come from a wide variety of backgrounds, but a significant number do so as qualified health professionals. There is a temptation to APL and credit existing knowledge of anatomy and physiology and then omit this subject from their course content. It is the experience of the teachers within the Education and Training group of the Reflexology Forum that this type of student not only benefits from working through this section of the curriculum, but also enjoys and appreciates the experience.

Tabular Format

An example of an anatomy and physiology exercise in tabular form is included in Table 14b. This format facilitates the investigation of a body system to whatever depth the student needs. Using this method has been found to enable students who have not studied the subject before to cover the subject satisfactorily. However, this can also be used by, for example, health professionals who have added fresh aspects to their understanding whilst revisiting their prior learning. Tabular format encourages concise, relevant statements of fact without the need to construct an essay type assignment. Care and time is needed to examine and analyse factual material to formulate short statements to fill the columns. The time and effort that previously had to be put in to produce an assignment of a required length can be applied to the extraction of information from the source material. However, some students will still wish to produce written assignments and this added home study will help their assimilation of the material. Experienced teachers will use a variety of techniques to facilitate student learning and the tabular format is offered as one tested method.

7.2 Overview of the Human Body

7.2.1 Cells, Tissues, Organs, Systems

Course content should cover the definitions of the terms: cell, tissue and organ and enable the student to understand how the cells combine to build tissue, the different types of which in turn form the variety of organs which are the component parts of the 11 body systems.

Table **7.1** contains the minimum required component parts of the systems of the body for this curriculum and is a useful overview of the subject.

7.2.2. Cell and Tissue – Structure and Function

Content relating to the cell structure should be limited to identifying membrane, cytoplasm, organelles and nucleus on a diagram.

Types of Cell

The student should be able to name the different types of blood cells and be able to identify the axon, neurone, myelin sheath and dendrite on a diagram of a typical nerve cell.

Cell function

Students should realise that the cell is the basic building block for all living organisms and each cell has specific functions. They must know the meaning of the terms diffusion, osmosis and the sodium pump, (active transport), but not be required to recount these processes in an examination. *However, there should be an appreciation of the significance of how these processes relate to the lymphatic system and disorders such as oedema.*

Students should understand that

- *the cell nucleus contains genetic information controlling the structure of the cell and how it functions*
- *cytoplasm is where chemical reactions, including cellular respiration, occur, enabling the cell to perform its functions*
- *the cell membrane acts as a barrier between the cell and its surroundings, controlling what substances can enter and leave the cell by diffusion, osmosis and active transport.*

Cell division

Students should know that new cells are formed from existing ones by the process of cell division. They should know that there are two types of cell division; mitosis and meiosis, and understand that mitosis occurs in growth and repair of all tissues (except nervous tissue, which once formed cannot repair or be replaced), and that meiosis occurs in the formation of gametes (eggs and sperm).

Students should understand that genetic mutations can occur during cell division and as a result of exposure to chemicals and radiation in the environment and that these mutations can result in the formation of tumours or in the inheritance of genetic disorders by offspring.

Tissue

Students should know that tissue is composed of a number of cells, identical in structure and function, held together by a matrix. Four different types of body tissue should be known as:

- Epithelial, forming covering and lining cell layers, e.g. in skin or the innermost layer of blood vessels/the gut.
- Muscular, contractile cells that bring about movement.
- Connective, joining tissues together to form organs or as packing between cells.
- Nervous, specialised to receive stimuli, transmit information and control muscle and gland action.

Organ

Students should know that an organ is made up of several different tissues working together to perform a major body function.

7.2.3 Homeostasis/Homeodynamics

Students should know the definition of the term homeostasis: That it was first coined by Walter Cannon from the Greek *homoios* – 'same' and *stasis* – 'standing' and refers to 'the body's ability to maintain a steady equilibrium within narrow limits'. As this equilibrium is continually being adjusted some authorities now prefer the term 'homeodynamics'.

Students should understand that body organs function most efficiently within narrow ranges of temperature, pH and body fluid concentration.

Stress and Feedback Systems

Students should know the widest definition of stress as being 'a stimulus that provides a response' but that stress is usually understood to mean more than usual stimulus or pressure. There should be understanding that the causes of stress can be exercise, fasting, fright, temperature changes, infection, disease and emotional disturbances/situations.

Also understanding the effects of stress upon homeodynamics is expected and the systems involved with the stress response, namely:

- *the short-term response mediated by the sympathetic nervous system and the adrenal medulla, resulting in elevated heart rate and blood pressure, dilation of bronchioles, elevation of blood glucose levels and depressed digestive activity.*
- *Long-term response in which the anterior pituitary gland releases ACTH, causing the adrenal cortex to release mineralocorticosteroids, which promote water and salt retention, resulting in increased blood volume which in turn raises blood pressure, and glucocorticosteroids, which increases blood glucose levels, promotes the conversion of fats and proteins to glucose and reduces both the inflammatory and immune responses.*

Students should know the definitions of the term 'negative feedback' as "the effector response to a stimulus negating or decreasing the effect of the original stimulus, restoring homeostasis", and 'positive feedback' as "a progressive amplification of a response caused by a stimulus, taking the body further away from a state of homeostasis". Students should be able to cite an example of each, e.g. negative feedback controlling body temperature and positive feedback controlling uterine contractions during labour.

Lifestyle and stress

There should be awareness of the effects of lifestyle upon the human organism. These lifestyle effects should be limited to environment, alcohol and drug abuse, smoking, extremes of diet, lack of exercise and stress (used as the term for tension, anxiety or worry).

7.2.4 Organisation of the human body

Students should be aware the body has a definite plan. They should be taught the *anatomical position* – standing erect, arms at the sides, eyes, toes and palms directed forward – and the importance of the latter to reflexology theory in that this changes the plotting of the zones.

Students should know importance to human structure of the anatomical directional terms (see Table 7.4) and be able to label these on a blank diagram.

7.3 System 1 – The Integumentary System
Components: Skin, Hair and Nails

The student should know the definition of the word integument as being 'covering'. Thus the integumentary system refers to the outer covering of the body often previously classified as just 'skin' but extends to include the nails and hair.

7.3.1 Skin

Structure

The student should be able to identify the component parts on a diagram of a cross section of skin including the epidermis, dermis, and fatty layer, nerves, sensory receptors, blood vessels, sebaceous glands and sweat glands.

Function

Students must be able to recall that the skin is the largest organ of the body and has the functions of protection, temperature control and excretion. Sensory receptors facilitate the sense of touch. How skin is maintained, repaired and replaced should be taught along with the mechanism of wound healing.

Skin and health

Students can revisit: Awareness of how disorders are evidenced via the skin in diabetes, liver, thyroid and circulatory problems. How sunlight stimulates production of melanin and the changes emotion, stress and shock can have upon the skin.

7.3.2 Hair

Structure

Students should know that hair is composed of protein – keratin, can be found on all parts of the body with the exception of palms of hands and soles of feet. Facts regarding rate of growth should be covered.

Function

Students should know that hair is for protection (for example, eyelashes protect the eye from foreign matter), temperature control, and sexual attraction.

7.3.3 Nails

Structure

The condition of the nail has significance in reflexology assessment thus students must know that nails are composed of the same protein as hair – keratin, hardened. They should be able to label the component parts of diagrams of a top view and cross section of the nail with the matrix, lunula, paronychium, eponychium, free edge, hyponychium, nail bed, fold, root and wall.

Function

Technical name – onyx. Functions of the nail should be known as protection of extra sensitive areas of toes and fingers and to assist fingers in grasping objects. Rate of growth is to replace every 5–6 months, fingernails growing faster than toenails and faster during the summer.

7.4 System 2 – The Respiratory System
Components: Naso-pharynx, Larynx, Trachea, Bronchi & Bronchioles and Lungs

The student should know that the purpose of the respiratory system is to take air into the lungs where oxygen is extracted into the blood stream to be taken to all body tissues where the cells can use it to produce energy. The by-product of this is carbon dioxide, which is returned to the lungs via the blood to be exchanged into waste air for exhalation.

Five stages of respiration
The five stages of respiration should be known: Ventilation, external respiration, transport of gases, internal respiration and cellular respiration

7.4.1 Structure

The student should be able to label on a diagram the following major components and associated structures: Nose, mouth, pharynx, larynx, trachea, bronchi, bronchioles, lungs, alveoli, parietal pleura, pleural cavity, visceral pleura, ribs, intercostals muscles and diaphragm.

Students should know that:
- The trachea is supported by C-shaped cartilage to prevent collapse and suffocation.
- There are three lobes to the right lung and two on the left.

7.4.2 Function

The fact that air is warmed, moistened and filtered by the upper structures of the system should be known. Students should understand that oxygen from the air is dissolved in the thin film of moisture on the cells lining the alveoli, it then diffuses through these cells and through the walls of the capillaries into the plasma of the blood. From the plasma it diffuses into the erythrocytes and combines with haemoglobin to form oxyhaemoglobin. In this way the blood can carry 70 times more oxygen than would be possible in a simple solution.

They should know the difference in composition of inspired and expired air:

Inspired	**Expired**
Oxygen: 21%	Oxygen: 16%
Carbon Dioxide: 0.04%	Carbon Dioxide: 4.5%

Nitrogen and Inert Gases remain the same; Water Vapour is variable

It should be understood that the mechanism of respiration consists of *Inspiration and Expiration*. This is brought about not by the lungs but by movement of the chest wall.

Inspiration is brought about by contraction of the diaphragm, which increases the depth of the thorax and contraction of the intercostal muscles which swing the ribs outwards and upwards and thus increases the diameter of the thorax.

Both these movements combine to increase the capacity of the thorax thus lowering the pressure within. As the air pressure is now greater outside the body, so air moves into the lungs.

Expiration is brought about by elastic recoil when the muscles relax and air is forced out as in a pair of bellows.

Students should be aware of the function of *mucus* as preventing the lining of the respiratory tract from drying out and trapping foreign particles for removal by the wafting action of tiny hair-like structures called *cilia*, and the possible implications of overproduction of mucus. They should also know the function of the pleural membranes as being a protective lining, enclosing the lungs and reducing friction between them and the chest wall.

Students should understand that smoking damages the respiratory system, paralysing cilia so that bacteria-laden mucus accumulates in the bronchi causing bronchitis. Constant coughing can rupture alveoli, causing emphysema. Tar in cigarette smoke is carcinogenic, causing lung cancer.

7.5 System 3 – The Cardiovascular System

Components: Heart, blood, blood vessels – arteries, veins, capillaries

The student should know that the cardiovascular system transports blood to and from all parts of the body and is essential to the maintenance of good health. Students should be aware of the different circuits of the system; systemic, pulmonary, portal/hepatic and foetal circulation and location and function of each.

7.5.1 Heart

Structure

Students should know that the heart is located below the sternum, 2/3 left of the midline of the body in the thoracic cavity and that its size is comparable to a man's closed fist. They must be able to label on a diagram the aorta, right and left atrium, right and left ventricle, tricuspid and bicuspid (mitral) valves, pulmonary and aortic valves, septum, superior and inferior vena cava. They should also be able to name the layers of heart wall from outside in as epicardium, myocardium and endocardium enclosed in the outer membrane the pericardium.

Students should understand the unique nature of cardiac muscle as being capable of constant contractions without fatigue and being able to contract without messages from the brain.

Students should understand that rate of heartbeat can be modified by the autonomic nervous system and by the hormone adrenaline.

Pulmonary circulation – structure

Students should be able to identify the component parts and describe the route taken by blood and the purpose of pulmonary circulation.

Heart – function

Students should know that the heart beats to pump blood through the miles of the body's blood vessels, that heart rate is 70–80 beats per minute on average at rest and is regulated by the vagus (10th cranial) nerve, and nerves from the autonomic nervous system.

7.5.2 The Blood

Composition

Knowledge that the blood is composed of plasma, red corpuscles or cells, (erythrocytes), that carry oxygen to the body cells, white corpuscles, (leucocytes), that destroy disease-causing micro-organisms and platelets that are much smaller than red cells and play a major part in clotting.

Function

Students should recall the primary functions of the blood as being:

- To transport water, oxygen, nutrients, enzymes and hormones to cells
- To carry away CO_2 and waste products to be eliminated through the lungs, skin, kidneys and large intestine.
- To help regulate body temperature.
- To help protect the body from infection via the action of leucocytes.
- To prevent blood loss via the action of platelets and clotting.

7.5.3 Blood vessels

The course will not require students to recall in examination the names of every blood vessel. Only those vessels that enter and leave the heart, lungs and liver, and those vessels that are normally used in the measurement of blood pressure or pulse, including the brachial, carotid and femoral arteries, and the primary vessels in the hand and wrist, ankle and foot, should be able to be recalled and identified on a blank diagram. However, during the coursework students should have completed diagrams of the complete vascular network.

Arteries

Students should know arteries carry blood away from the heart, have thick elastic walls to manage the high pressure from the heartbeat, are controlled by the autonomic nervous system and supplied with Pacinian sensory receptors that monitor blood pressure. Arterioles are small arteries that carry blood to the capillaries. Arterioles in the skin help regulate body temperature by widening when the body is too hot, allowing more blood to enter surface capillaries to be cooled.

Capillaries

Students should know that capillaries are microscopic vessels composed of a single layer of cells that connect arterioles and venules. Their function is to allow passage of nutrients and waste between blood and cells within tissues and organs.

Veins

They should know veins carry blood back to the heart, are much thinner walled and nearer to the surface than arteries and have valves to prevent backflow of blood as it is under less pressure than in the arteries. Venules are small veins that connect to capillaries.

Students should know the connection of the functions of the spleen and liver that relate to the cardiovascular system, namely:
- *That the liver produces plasma proteins that give blood its thickness and help in the clotting process.*
- *That the Kupffer cells in the liver break down worn out red blood cells and destroy bacteria.*
- *That the liver stores iron from broken down red blood cells.*
- *That the liver stores blood that is not in the general circulation.*
- *The spleen stores blood not in the general circulation.*
- *The spleen contains T- and B- lymphocyte white blood cells which are activated by the presence of disease organisms to bring about an immune response.*
- *The spleen and liver are important sites of red blood cell formation in foetuses and that the spleen can fulfil this function in adults in times of need.*
- *The spleen can break down old, worn-out red blood cells.*

7.5.4 Blood pressure

Students should understand:
- How blood pressure is measured using a sphygmomanometer.
- *That blood pressure is controlled short-term by the cardiovascular centre (CVC), in the medulla and pons of the brain, acting on information received from baroreceptors (pressure receptors), and chemoreceptors (sensitive to carbon dioxide levels in blood), in the walls of the aortic arch and carotid arteries, and by circulating hormones. In response to this input, the CVC brings about vasodilation or vasoconstriction, plus changes in heart rate and stroke volume.*

Students should be able to describe how the kidneys are involved in the long-term control of blood pressure by:
- *Regulating blood volume.*
- *The Renin-angiotensin-aldosterone system.*

They should be aware of the factors that affect blood pressure:
- The force of blood as it is pumped from the left ventricle
- The volume of blood in the system
- The resistance to the blood flow in the arteries

Students should know the definitions, and understand the mechanism, of the following:
- Blood Pressure: The force of blood measured on artery walls

- Systolic: BP during ventricular contraction – highest BP
- Diastolic: BP during ventricular relaxation – lowest BP
- Pulse: The wave of blood felt as each heartbeat is pumped
- Blood shunting: the transfer of blood volume to an area of the body where it is required e.g. from digestive organs to lungs and muscles when a sudden need for activity occurs
- Varicose veins: dilated veins with a backflow of blood usually caused by the dysfunction of vein valves

The recall of numerical data for the cardiovascular system is confined to approximate normal systolic and diastolic measurements for young, adult and elderly men and women.

(The recommendation is made that students who aspire to practise reflexology at a clinical level should be able to use a sphygmomanometer to record BP before and following a treatment. The resulting evidence that treatment reduces hypertension, raises the BP of hypotensive clients and has little effect on normal BP will be invaluable proof of the normalising aspect of reflexology.)

7.6 System 4 – The Lymphatic System

Components: Lymph fluid, lymph vessels, lymph nodes (organs), lymph nodules, thoracic duct, lymphatic duct, spleen, thymus and tonsils

The student should understand that the lymphatic system is a subsidiary circulatory system that also reaches parts of the body not covered by blood vessels, with the exception of the CNS, bone, cartilage and teeth. It connects with the vascular system in that whilst whole blood remains inside the blood vessels, part of the blood permeates through the capillary walls into the tissue spaces becoming interstitial fluid. This tissue fluid bathes the cells trading its nutrients for the waste products of metabolism and is absorbed into the lymph vessels to be filtered and detoxified as it passes through lymph nodes before being eventually drained back into the blood via two ducts in the upper thorax.

Function
Students should be able to recount the primary functions of the lymphatic system:
- To carry excess fluid and foreign particles from the body tissues and cells.
- To transport fats from the digestive tract to the blood.
- To produce lymphocytes to deal with waste and toxins that builds up in the cells.
- To develop antibodies to defend the body against infection.

They should know the definition of antibody to be a protein produced by the body to protect against an antigen, and an antigen to be a substance that when introduced into the body causes it to produce an antibody.

7.6.1 Lymph fluid – structure

It should be understood that lymph is a colourless fluid derived from blood plasma created when it filters through the capillary wall into the tissue spaces. It is the excess tissue fluid that cannot re-enter the blood at capillaries, but drains into blind-ending lymphatic capillaries. Lymph consists of plasma substances such as fibrinogen, serum

Anatomy & Physiology

albumin and serum globulin, water and infection fighting lymphocytes, waste products, e.g. carbon dioxide and urea, fats absorbed from the diet and bacteria and cell debris.

7.6.2 Lymph vessels – structure

Students should know that there are lymph capillaries which are thin-walled, permeable vessels running alongside both arteries and veins into which tissue fluid passes. Molecules too large to pass through blood capillary walls can get through lymph vessel walls to be carried away into larger vessels called lymphatics provided with valves to prevent backflow. The largest lymph vessels end with the thoracic duct that drains lymph arriving from all the body, except the upper right quadrant, into the left subclavian (innominate) vein back into the bloodstream. The lymph from the right side of the head, neck, thorax and arm drains through the right lymphatic duct into the right subclavian (innominate) vein.

7.6.3 Lymph nodes and Lymph Nodules

Structure

Students should know lymph nodes and lymph nodules are all over the body and be able to draw on an outline diagram of the human body these structures, nodes and glands: The tonsils, thoracic duct, cisterna chyli, lymphatic duct, thymus, axillary nodes, mammary lymphatics, spleen, Peyer's patches and inguinal lymph nodes.

Students should also be taught the difference between nodes and nodules: Lymph nodes (also known as glands) are masses of lymphatic tissue surrounded by a connective tissue capsule and have lymph vessels delivering lymph to them. Nodules have neither and are small and solitary with the exception of tonsils and Peyer's patches.

Function

They should understand that lymph nodes and nodules are where lymphocytes are produced and concentrated to detoxify the lymph fluid and fight infection.

Tonsils

There should be understanding that there is a ring of lymphoid tissue around the entrance to the food and air passages: the adenoid or pharyngeal tonsil, the palatine tonsil and the lingual tonsil, which react to, ingested substances that pose a threat to health. They produce antibodies for local infection and lymphocytes for immunity.

Peyer's Patches

Students should know that Peyer's patches are large clusters of lymph nodules found in the ileum, lower part of the small intestine

Major lymph organs – spleen and thymus

Spleen

The spleen should be understood to be the largest lymph mass which acts as a filter for worn out red blood cells, abnormal cells and selectively filters white cells and platelets. It produces antibodies that immobilise foreign particles and stores blood for release in emergency.

Thymus

The mass of lymph tissue behind the sternum should be understood to be the thymus which is more active before puberty to control growth as an endocrine gland but its lymphatic function is to process lymphocytes to become active 'T'cells, vital to the immune system.

7.6.4 Autoimmunity

Students should also know that:

- the lymphatic system has a role in acquiring immunity from infection.
- the meaning of 'autoimmune' as the development of an immune response against one's own body cells.
- how allergies may be triggered and the way the body responds.

Infection

The student should be able to recognise the significance of swollen glands, swollen oedemic lower limbs and the formation of pus during infection and be aware that they can be the result of many different conditions which may indicate a reflexology contraindication (see Appendix 3).

Intersystem relationship

Recall of chemical formulae will not be required, but the relationship between the lymphatic system and the nervous, cardiovascular and endocrine systems should be understood.

7.7 System 5 – The Digestive System

Components: Mouth, teeth, tongue, salivary glands, oesophagus, cardiac sphincter, stomach, pyloric sphincter, small intestines (duodenum, jejunum, ileum), illeocaecal sphincter, appendix, large intestines (colon), rectum, anus, *accessory organs*; liver, pancreas, gall bladder

Students should demonstrate understanding of the way food is essential for energy and the maintenance of good health and knowledge of the processes food undergoes as it passes through the alimentary canal and is acted upon by the digestive accessory organs. They should be able to recall the three basic categories of food (carbohydrates, fats and proteins), and vitamins, minerals, evaluate the importance of good diet.

Important limitation

Each student should be informed that, although the training covers detailed information of the nature and importance of diet, this training is not in nutrition and he/she will not be a qualified dietician.

7.7.1 The alimentary canal

Location and structure

The course should equip the student to draw and label on a blank outline of the human body various structures of the alimentary canal and describe the important features of each structure as follows:

- Mouth – lips, teeth – canine, incisors, premolars and molars, tongue, salivary glands and epiglottis
- the oesophagus
- cardiac sphincter, the stomach and pyloric sphincter
- 17ft of small intestine (the three sections being-duodenum, jejunum and ileum)
- the appendix, the ileocecal valve (sphincter)
- 5ft of large intestines (colon).

As there are related reflex points and areas, students must be able to recall the structure of the colon to be caecum, ascending colon, hepatic flexure, transverse colon, splenic flexure, descending colon, sigmoid flexure, rectum and anus.

Function
The functions of the components of the alimentary canal should be understood to be:

Mouth – lips
Mouth – lips: to take in food and drink and keep it in that area whilst digestion starts.

Teeth
Teeth – canine, incisors, premolars and molars: to bite and separate, rip, crush and chew food to commence breakdown for easier action by enzymes.

Tongue and epiglottis
Tongue – facilitate taste and form the masticated food into a bolus for easy passage down the canal where the epiglottis prevents it entering the air passage (trachea).

Salivary glands
The salivary glands secrete saliva (ptyalin) that contains the enzyme amylase to commence breakdown of carbohydrate.

Oesophagus
The oesophagus moves the bolus down toward the stomach by the action of peristalsis and the cardiac sphincter opens to allow the bolus to enter the stomach, closes to prevent the hydrochloric gastric acid escaping upward, and 'burn' the oesophagus.

Stomach
In the stomach digestion commences on protein and hours later food passes into the duodenum where enzymes from the pancreas and microvilli in the small intestine, together with bile produced by the liver and stored in the gall bladder, are added to the food to further breakdown carbohydrate, protein and fat.

Small intestine
Whilst the simplified food is slowly passed through the rest of the small intestine by peristalsis it is digested into its simplest form and absorption of these nutrients into the bloodstream commences, (with the exception of fats, which are absorbed into the lymphatic system at the ileum).

Appendix

Though traditionally thought to be without function the appendix wall contains many lymphatic nodules with probable immune system value.

Ileocecal valve (sphincter)

The ileocecal sphincter prevents backflow into the ileum of the contents of the colon.

Colon, rectum, anus

Before it is passed out through the rectum and anal sphincter the waste remaining from undigested food is slowly passed through the large intestine (colon) and has most of the water content removed via absorption through the colon walls, being coloured by bile pigment and becoming solid faecal matter.

7.7.2 Accessory digestive organs

Liver

Each student should know that the liver is the largest internal organ, weighing about 3lbs, comprises 2 lobes, the right being six times larger than the left, each lobe being made up of many lobules containing plates of hepatic cells that produce bile.

Students could revisit the following toward the end of their training: Between the plates are sinusoids that supply O_2 and nutrients and which contain Kupffer cells that remove bacteria, foreign matter and worn out blood cells. Students should be taught that the liver has many chemical functions:

- *produces bile to breakdown fat*
- *synthesises clotting factors from amino acids*
- *deactivates amino acids and converts simple sugars*
- *stores various fat and water soluble vitamins, iron and copper*
- *synthesises vitamin A from carotene*
- *detoxicates drugs and noxious substances*
- *metabolises ethanol in alcohol*
- *inactivates hormones*
- *desaturates fat*
- *produces heat*

Recall of all of these functions would not be expected in examination, though a substantial proportion would evidence understanding.

Gall bladder

The student should be able to explain that the gall bladder stores and concentrates bile to pass down the common bile duct to break down fat in the small intestine.

Pancreas

Apart from its endocrine (ductless) function, the pancreas has the exocrine task of passing pancreatic juice containing enzymes through the pancreatic duct which joins the common bile duct to act upon carbohydrate, protein and fat in the small intestine.

7.7.3 Digestive timing

The knowledge and recall of timing of digestion is limited to:
- *Within 1 minute with saliva acting on carbohydrate in the mouth.*
- *Food stays from 1½–4 hours in the stomach.*
- *2–4 hours in the small intestine.*
- *10 hours to several days in the large intestine.*

7.7.4 Chemistry of digestion

Knowledge of the chemistry of the digestive process is limited to:
- Food is composed of carbohydrate, protein and fat.
- *On a simple chart of enzyme action the student should be able to insert in its correct place and sequence the following terms and enzymes:*
  - i. *The enzyme amylase (in ptyalin) acts on polysaccharides (cooked starch); amylase converts polysaccharides to disaccharides in the mouth and small intestine; the enzymes sucrase, maltase and lactase convert disaccharides to monosaccharides (e.g. glucose) in the ileum.*
  - ii. *The enzyme pepsin converts proteins to peptones in the stomach; the enzymes trypsin and chymotrypsin convert peptones to polypeptides and polypeptides to amino acids in the duodenum; the peptidase enzymes convert polypeptides into amino acids in the ileum.*
  - iii. *Pancreatic lipase enzyme and bile salts emulsify fats; lipase converts fats to fatty acids and glycerol. (See section A3.6 in Appendix 3 for example chart.)*
- Knowledge of the pH condition throughout the alimentary canal is limited to the stomach being strongly acidic and this being neutralised in the small intestine.

7.7.5 Nutrition, vitamins and minerals

Students should have a basic understanding of how nutrients and a balanced diet promote and maintain good health. The knowledge of vitamins and minerals should be limited to the following with a fundamental understanding of their impact upon health. Knowledge of which vitamins and minerals can be unsafe if the normal dose is exceeded should be: Vitamins A, B1, B3, B6, B12, C, D, E. Minerals: Calcium, Magnesium, Iron, Iodine, Potassium, and Sodium.

Students should be aware that modern farming and food processing has an effect upon the food we eat and may affect the body's ability to maintain good health.

Prescription and opinion

Each student shall be aware that this qualification will enable them to prescribe reflexology only. They should take care to present advice on diet and nutrition in the form of a suggestion or opinion and only when there is evidence of real need, in which case a referral to a qualified nutrition counsellor or dietician would be appropriate. Where reflexologists hold a qualification in nutrition there are valid reasons for presenting such advice as a different session, even immediately following a treatment, as is the case all multi-disciplined practitioners. 'Wearing one hat at a time' and having well-defined boundaries is advantageous for both practitioner and client, involving issues such as consent, taking responsibility, client/public perception, practitioner's income and acknowledging one's own limitations.

Any significant change in lifestyle advised on a first treatment could make the evaluation of the benefits of starting reflexology more difficult to ascertain and students should be taught the advantages of introducing any changes gradually.

Drinking water after treatment

The above can apply to the advice to drink water. Generally this is very good advice. Public awareness of this is greater now than ever before and it may be that the client already drinks the recommended amount. Experienced reflexologists have reported that water following a treatment reduces the incidence of any unpleasant reactions to reflexology and offering a client a glass seems good practice and a pleasant conclusion to a treatment. This is not the same as prescribing excessive daily amounts of water to 'flush away the toxins' from which the client may report increased micturition mistakenly attributed to improved kidney efficiency, or a rogue symptom.

7.8 System 6 – The Urinary (Renal) System

Components: Kidneys, ureters, urinary bladder, urethra, urine

The student should understand that the Urinary or Renal system has the principal function of filtering waste products from the blood through the left and right kidneys, processing these into urine. This fluid is passed via gravity and peristalsis through the two ureter tubes that converge into the urinary bladder where it is stored until it is convenient to expel it by muscular action through the urethra.

7.8.1 Urinary system – Location and structure

The student should be able to draw and identify the component parts (left & right kidneys, ureters, bladder and urethra) on a blank body outline and briefly describe the size and gross structure of each part.

Kidney and ureter structure and function

The understanding of the structure and function of the kidneys is limited to being bean-shaped, 10–15 cm (4–5 inches) in length with an outer cortex and inner medulla that contains millions of filter tubes called nephrons which filter excess water, salts and urea from the blood as it passes through. The location of the right kidney being slightly lower than the left should be known. The knowledge that the ureters are narrow muscular tubes about eleven inches long to carry urine from the kidneys by gravity and peristaltic action to the bladder is sufficient. Students should know that filtration of the blood by the nephrons occurs by a process called "ultra-filtration", which is brought about by the high pressure of blood flowing through the kidneys.

As osmosis is the process by which water is reabsorbed from urine back into the bloodstream in the kidneys, (under the control of the hormone ADH), students should be able to recount the definition of osmosis as being 'the passage of water through a semi-permeable membrane'.

Bladder and urethra structure and function

The understanding of the structure and function of the bladder is limited to its capacity of storing usually 300–500 ml (1 pint) of urine before sensory receptors instigate expulsion of urine by muscular contraction of the bladder walls and opening of its sphincter. The urethra should be noted as being 4 cm (1½ inches) in the average female and approximately 20 cm (8 inches) in men.

7.8.2 Fluid balance and composition of urine

Under normal circumstances the output of urine is directly related to the intake of fluid. The student should know the constituents of urine and how these vary with diet and temperature.

Regulation of blood pressure

Students should be able to describe <u>briefly</u> how the Renin-angiotensin-aldosterone system in the kidneys affects blood pressure.

7.9 System 7 – The Endocrine System

Components: Pituitary gland, hypothalamus, pineal gland, thyroid gland, parathyroid glands, thymus, adrenal glands, pancreas (islets of Langerhans), gonads – ovaries & testes, hormones

- Students should understand the term endocrine means 'ductless' and refers to the system of glands that secrete hormones, chemical messengers, directly (not via ducts) into the bloodstream to be quickly transported to target glands or other sites of operation to control metabolism and a wide variety of body processes.
- They should be able to draw and identify the component glands listed above on a blank outline of the human body.
- *They should also be able to evaluate the interrelationship between this system and the nervous system.*

7.9.1 The pituitary gland – structure and function

The understanding of the pituitary (or *hypophysis*) should be limited to: its being called the 'master' gland because of the control of its hormones over so many of the other endocrine glands. That it has two lobes, anterior and posterior and, being no larger than a pea, is located centrally at the base of the brain. Students should be able to recall the hormones produced or stored by each lobe and name its target site and resulting action (see Table 7.9.1 overleaf).

Hypothalamus

Students should understand that the hypothalamus is not actually classified as an endocrine gland but is part of the nervous system, an area of the brain near the pituitary gland. However, it is so linked with the pituitary by nerves and blood vessels and essential to endocrine function that it is considered along with this system.

Table 7.9.1

Hormone	Abbreviation	Target site	Action
The **anterior** lobe produces these hormones:			
Thyroid stimulating hormone	TSH	Thyroid Gland	Thyroxin
Adrenocorticotrophic hormone	ACTH	Adrenal glands	Cortisone
Somatotrophin or growth hormone	GH	All body cells	General growth
Follicle stimulating hormone	FSH	Ovaries	Oestrogen
		or Testes	Sperm
Luteinising hormone	LH	Ovaries	Progesterone
		or Testes	Testosterone
Prolactin	PRL	Mammary glands	Lactation
Melanocyte stimulating hormone	MSH	Skin, melanocytes	Dispersal of melanin
The **posterior** lobe stores these hormones produced by the Hypothalamus:			
Vasopressin, antidiuretic hormone	ADH	Kidneys/arteries	Decrease of urine
Oxytocin		Uterus	Induces labour
		Breasts	Stimulates milk

7.9.2 The pineal gland/body

Students should know the structure of the pineal gland as limited to its small size and location as being central in, and at the rear of, the brain. Recall should be that it primarily secretes *melatonin* into the blood in relation to the amount of light entering the eyes – daylight inhibiting its release. Although all the functions of the pineal body are not understood some facts that students should be able to link this gland are the release of melatonin to inhibiting puberty, affecting mood and causing depression, and regulating the body clock or diurnal rhythms affecting sleep and appetite. The students should be made aware of the links with 'jet lag' and SAD (seasonal affective disorder).

7.9.3 The Thyroid gland

The students' knowledge of the thyroid gland should extend to that two lobes lie on each side of the trachea and it is responsible for regulating the metabolic rate in the body. During the course the student should gain understanding of the effect these hormones have both in health and illness. Especially thyroxine, which if over produced causes hyperthyroidism, increased metabolic rate and, conversely, hypothyroidism when under produced. ***Students should be able to recount the symptoms of both of the above states, which will be covered in section 8 – the Disorders or reflexology and ill health***

Thyroid hormones:
- Thyroxine – T_4
- Triiodothyronine – T_3 Both control metabolism of foods, in the presence of oxygen in cells, into energy; growth, development and proper functioning of systems such as the nervous, skeletal and reproductive
- Calcitonin – Acts on bone and kidneys to regulate calcium levels

In examination recall will be limited to generalised understanding of the effects which thyroid hormones have on which systems, namely: Thyroxine and triiodothyronine speed up metabolism, growth and development and calcitonin lowers blood calcium levels by promoting its uptake by bones and teeth.

7.9.4 The Parathyroid Glands

Knowledge of the four parathyroid glands will be limited to understanding their location on the posterior surface of the thyroid with which they work to regulate blood calcium levels. Students should know this is a negative feedback mechanism and recall that the only hormone involved is:

- Parathyroid Hormone (PTH) or parathormone. Acts in a variety of ways to raise calcium levels in the blood.

Knowledge that PTH reduces phosphorous and activates Vitamin D is also useful showing links to problems with bones, muscle spasm (tetany) and nerve transmission.

7.9.5 Thymus

Knowledge of the thymus gland will be limited to the location of its two lobes being behind the sternum, that it has both endocrine and lymphatic functions. Students should be able to describe the functions of the thymus as the following:

- That its work in regulating growth is accomplished before puberty, it reduces in size in adults becoming connective tissue in old age.
- The lymphatic function of the thymus starts before birth when stem cells migrate to it from the bone marrow and liver to multiply and differentiate thus producing 'T' (thymus) lymphocytes (T-cells).
- Thymosin is a hormone secreted by the thymus. It stimulates maturation of T-cells in the thymus.

7.9.6 The Adrenal glands

Structure

Each student should understand the importance, especially in reflexology, of the adrenal glands and that they have 50 functions. The student should be able to locate these on the top of each kidney accounting for their other name – the suprarenal glands. Students should be able to recall their structure to be an inner medulla encased by the outer cortex, each area having distinct functions. Students should be able to demonstrate their understanding of the functions of the adrenal cortex and medulla as:

Function

Adrenal Cortex:
- Secretes 3 hormone groups:
  1. Glucocorticoids: recall limited to hormones Cortisone and Cortisol involvement in metabolism and response to stress. Especially suppressing inflammation and response to allergy
  2. Minralocorticoids: recall limited to hormone Aldosterone and the regulation of fluid balance and blood pressure. Students should be aware of the rennin-angiotensin-aldosterone response between the adrenals and the kidneys
  3. Sex hormones: Recall limited to the comparatively insignificant amounts of Androgens (male/female) and Progesterone/oestrogen (female) hormones

Adrenal Medulla:

- Secretes 2 hormones – Adrenaline, (Epinephrine), and Noradrenaline: Recall limited to ratio <u>80% Adrenaline : 20% Noradrenaline</u>, that they augment the *sympathetic ANS* (see nervous system) in the *'fight or flight'* response to *stress*.

The student should be able to demonstrate understanding of the rapid involvement of the <u>ANS</u> and <u>adrenal medulla</u> in response to short term stressors and the slower response of the <u>ANS</u> and <u>adrenal cortex</u> to long-term stressors.

7.9.7 The Pancreas

The student's knowledge of the pancreas will extend to its location as being left upper abdomen, behind the stomach, having a 'head body and tail' and that it has both endocrine and exocrine functions. Its digestive exocrine (through a duct) properties are considered in section 7.6.3.

The student should be able to recall that the three endocrine hormones of the pancreas are contained in the <u>islets of Langerhans</u> and be able to link their names with the processes below:

- <u>Glucagon</u>: Acts on the liver to release and produce more glucuose. Glucagon is released by pancreas when glucose level in the blood is reduced (e.g. during fasting) and is inhibited when blood sugar is high.
- <u>Insulin</u>: Importantly, acts to reduce blood glucose levels but also has an effect on fat and protein metabolism. The pancreas releases insulin when blood sugar (glucose) levels rise and inhibited when they fall.
- <u>Somatostatin</u>: Same hormone as GHRIH from Hypothalamus but when secreted from the pancreas it inhibits glucagon, insulin and pancreatic enzymes.

7.9.8 The Gonads

The student should know that the primary reproductive organs, the gonads, are the testes (male) and ovaries (female) and are included in this system too because of their endocrine function. The extent of recall for this is to link the hormones below with their functions.

Female hormones
- <u>Oestrogen</u>: Controls female secondary sex characteristics, promotes repair of the uterus lining after menstruation and development of ova in the ovaries
- <u>Progesterone</u>: Controls thickening of the uterus lining in preparation for implantation of the embryo, maintains the uterus lining during the first three months of pregnancy and stops release of eggs from the ovaries.

Male hormones
- <u>Testosterone</u>: Controls male secondary sex characteristics and promotes development of sperm in the testes.

7.10 System 8 – The Reproductive System

Components: Female – Vulva, vagina, uterus, fallopian (uterine) tubes, ovaries, ova and breasts (mammary glands. Male – Testes, vas deferens, prostate gland, sperm, penis

ore Curriculum for Reflexology in the United Kingdom

7.10.1 The Female Organs

Students should know that the female reproductive organs, or genitalia, are divided into external and internal organs and accessory glands.

External genitalia

The external genitalia are known collectively as the *vulva*, and students should demonstrate recall that the vulva consists of:
- Labia majora
- Labia minora
- Clitoris
- Vestibule
- Hymen
- Greater vestibular glands

Students should be aware of the functions of the female external genitalia and be able to label their location on a given diagram.

Internal genitalia

Students must be able to describe structure and function of the following internal genitalia, and label them on a given diagram.

It is expected that students should know that the internal organs of the female reproductive system lie in the pelvic cavity and consist of the vagina, cervix, uterus, two fallopian tubes, (oviducts) and two ovaries.

Vagina

The student should be able to demonstrate knowledge of the following structures and their functions, limited to:

Vagina is a fibromuscular tube lined with stratified epithelium, connecting the external and internal organs of reproduction. It also serves as a passageway for menstrual blood, forms part of the birth canal during labour, and is the site of penetration and release of semen during intercourse. It runs up and back at an angle of about 45 degrees between the bladder in front and rectum and anus behind. Stratified squamous epithelium lines the inside, forming ridges or rugae.

The vagina has no secretory glands but the surface is kept moist by cervical secretions. Between puberty and menopause Lactobacillus Acidophilus microbes are normally present and they secrete lactic acid, maintaining the pH between 4.9 and 3.5. The acidity inhibits the growth of most microbes that may enter the vagina from the perineum.

Uterus

Uterus is a hollow muscular pear-shaped organ. It lies in the pelvic cavity between the urinary bladder and the rectum. The walls of the uterus are composed of three layers of tissue, which respond to hormonal secretions. The innermost lining of the uterus, (endometrium), thickens every month ready to act as a nourishing bed for the fertilised

Anatomy & Physiology

69

ovum. The top of the uterus opens out into fallopian tubes which lead to the ovaries, and the bottom end, called the cervix, opens into the vagina, forming the birth canal.

Knowledge of the function of the uterus is limited to being the place where the foetus grows and develops. Every month it prepares itself for possible pregnancy, and if there is no fertilisation, menstruation occurs (explained later). The uterus has layers of tissue that expand during pregnancy to accommodate a foetus.

Fallopian Tubes
Structure
Fallopian tubes are two long, funnel shaped tubes which have an outer covering of ligament, a middle layer of smooth muscle and are lined with ciliated epithelium. They start at the top of the uterus and extend outwards, close to the ovaries. The end of each tube has finger-like projections which lie very close to the ovary, to catch an egg when ovulation takes place.

Function
The fallopian tubes, also called uterine tubes or oviducts, are a passageway from the ovaries to the uterus for the ovum, as well as the site of fertilisation. Sperm swim up these tubes to reach the ovum, and fertilisation takes place in the tubes.

Ovaries
Structure
Ovaries are the female gonads, or glands; are almond-shaped, and are positioned either side of the uterus, just below the fallopian tubes. They are attached to the uterus by a ligament.

Functions
The ovaries secrete hormones, progesterone and oestrogen, whose functions are described in section 7.9.8 (endocrine system). They also store female sexual cells called ova or eggs (singular: ovum). Ova exist in the body at birth but are undeveloped and called follicles. After puberty, one follicle develops to maturity and ruptures, releasing a mature ovum every month. This is known as ovulation. Ovulation allows the possibility of fertilisation or menstruation.

Ovum
Structure
Students should know that an ovum is a female germ cell or egg. It forms by a cell division called meiosis in the ovaries. Each ovum is spherical in shape and has a nucleus containing 23 chromosomes, half the number found in all other body cells. The nucleus is surrounded by cytoplasm containing yolk, which feeds the fertilised egg during its journey to the uterus. The cytoplasm is surrounded by a cell membrane, which toughens after a sperm has entered, preventing other sperm from getting in.

Accessory Glands
Breasts or Mammary Glands
Students should be able to demonstrate awareness that the breasts or mammary glands are accessory glands of the female reproductive system. In the female the breasts are quite small until puberty, and they also exist in the male but only in a rudimentary form.

Students should know the structure and function of the breasts: The breasts consist of glandular tissue, fibrous and fatty tissue. Glandular tissue forms lobes, which open into several ducts. The ducts open onto the surface of the nipple. In pregnancy the lobes develop and produce milk under the control of the anterior pituitary gland hormone prolactin. There are numerous sensory nerve endings in the nipple, and as they are stimulated by the baby sucking, impulses pass to the hypothalamus and the flow of the hormone oxytocin (from the posterior pituitary gland), is increased, promoting the release of milk.

Function
The mammary glands are active only during pregnancy and after the birth of a baby when they produce milk.

7.10.2 The Male Organs

The students should be able to describe the structure and functions of the following components of the male reproductive system: Testes, vas deferens, prostate gland, sperm, penis.

Testes
The testes are the reproductive glands of the male and are the equivalent of the ovaries in the female.

Structure
The testes are two glands contained within a sac of deeply pigmented skin, fibrous and connective tissue and smooth muscle called the scrotum. They develop in the abdomen before descending into the scrotum just before birth. They sit either side of the penis.

Function
The testes produce spermatozoa (sperm) and the male sex hormone testosterone that is responsible for male sexual characteristics. Sperm develop in the testes and are stored in the epididymis, which opens into the vas deferens. Sperm must be kept at a slightly lower temperature than the average body temperature.

Vas Deferens/Spermatic Cords
Structure and functions
Two spermatic cords suspend each testis in the scrotum. They are composed of blood and lymph vessels, nerves and a deferent duct (vas deferens). The epididymis, a tightly coiled tube, opens from the top of each testis and then straightens out to form the deferent duct, called the vas deferens. The epididymis stores sperm before being transported to the vas deferens. The sperm then travel up and into the urethra, which runs through the centre of the penis, for deposit into the vagina during intercourse. The vas deferens has muscular walls, helping to push the sperm forward into the penis.

Prostate Gland
Structure and functions
The prostate gland lies in the pelvic cavity in front of the rectum and behind the symphysis pubis, surrounding the first part of the urethra. It consists of an outer fibrous covering,

a layer of smooth muscle and glandular substance composed of columnar epithelial cells. It secretes two types of thin lubricating fluid that passes into the urethra through numerous ducts. One type helps keep the lining of the urethra moist, and the other is part of the seminal fluid, which activates the swimming action of, and nourishes the sperm, helping them travel along the urethra into the female.

Penis

Structure

The penis is the main external sex organ of the male. It has three important parts: the erectile tissue, the foreskin and the urethra. The penis consists of three bodies of spongy, erectile tissue all running lengthways. Two of these run side by side and above the urethra (tube running through centre of penis which acts as a transporter for either sperm or urine) and one lies underneath forming a tube containing the urethra which becomes the tip of the penis, known as the "glans". The tissue is full of blood vessels. Surrounding the glans is the prepuce, or foreskin, a loose double fold of skin which protects the glans.

Function

The penis has two roles. The first is as an organ of excretion, carrying urine from the bladder for excretion. The second is as an organ of reproduction, during sexual activity becoming filled with blood and therefore rigid to allow for penetration into the vagina of the female, and consequently safe delivery of semen (sperm and fluid).

Sperm

A spermatozoon, (spermatozoa pl.), is a male germ cell, which forms by the cell division called meiosis. Each one has a head (male sex cell), a middle section and a tail that helps to propel the sperm towards the ovum. Each head has 23 chromosomes. A sperm fertilises the ovum by inserting its head into the ovum, and the tail then degenerates. Only one sperm is needed to fertilise one ovum, but semen (the fluid ejaculated through the penis in intercourse) contains millions of sperm to heighten the chances of fertilisation.

7.10.3 Conception

The student must be able to describe the process of conception, and in turn the process of menstruation when conception does not occur. *They must understand the process of Negative Feedback (explained under menstruation).*

Conception is the formation of an embryo as a result of an ovum being fertilised by a sperm in the fallopian tubes.

Males and females produce specialised reproductive germ cells, called *gametes.* In the male they are called spermatozoa and in the female, ova. The gametes contain the genetic material or genes, on *chromosomes,* which pass on to the next generation. In other body cells there are 46 chromosomes arranged in 23 pairs, but in the gametes there are only 23, one from each pair. Gametes are formed by meiosis. When the ovum is fertilised by a sperm, the result is called a *zygote.* The zygote then contains 23 pairs of chromosomes, one of each pair obtained from the father and one from the mother. The zygote then undergoes many mitotic cell divisions to form an ever increasingly large ball of cells called an embryo, which is moved along the fallopian tubes towards the uterus by the wafting action of the ciliated epithelium lining the fallopian tubes, and by the contraction of the smooth muscles in the walls of the fallopian tubes. When the embryo arrives at the uterus it embeds itself in the lining layer, called the endometrium, in a process called implantation. Part of the embryo develops into the placenta, part into the foetus and the rest develops into the amniotic sac around the foetus. The foetus grows and develops during the 40-week gestation period before birth.

Hormones involved in conception

Students should be able to show knowledge and understanding of the roles of female reproductive hormones involved in the menstrual cycle.

In alternate ovaries each month, FSH (follicle stimulating hormone) from the anterior pituitary in the brain, stimulates maturation of a follicle (the immature egg in the ovary, and causes the maturing follicle lining cells to produce increasing amounts of the hormone oestrogen, which also helps stimulate maturation of the follicle into an ovum. When a certain level of oestrogen is present in the blood, the hypothalamus secretes LHRH (Luteinising Hormone Releasing Hormone) that stimulates the anterior pituitary to secrete LH (Luteinising Hormone). High levels of oestrogen and LH together trigger ovulation, in which the follicle migrates to the edge of the ovary and ruptures its wall, releasing of the mature follicle, now called an ovum. As soon as ovulation occurs, the lining cells of the (now empty) follicle are stimulated by the presence of LH to develop into the corpus luteum (yellow body), which secretes progesterone. Progesterone helps the lining of the uterus become thicker and the glands in the uterus produce increased amounts of watery mucus. This is believed to assist the passage of the sperm through the uterus to the uterine tubes where the ovum is fertilised. There is similar increase in the secretion of watery mucus by the glands of the fallopian tubes and by cervical glands that lubricate the vagina. An ovum can only survive in fertilisable form for a very short time after ovulation, maybe as little as 8 hours. The sperm, deposited during intercourse in the vagina, may be capable of fertilisation only for about 24–72 hours.

If the ovum is fertilised, it forms a single cell called a zygote, which undergoes successive cell divisions by mitosis to form a ball of cells called an embryo. Once the embryo has implanted in the lining of the uterus it starts to produce Human Chorionic Gonadotrophin (HCG) hormone, which enables the corpus luteum to remain intact, continue producing progesterone so that the zygote can remain embedded in the uterus, and so that no other follicles in the ovaries become mature. During this time the placenta develops and gradually takes over the production of progesterone from the corpus luteum, after about 3 to 4 months.

7.10.4 Menstruation

Students must understand the process of menstruation: If the ovum is not fertilised, no HCG hormone is produced, so the corpus luteum slowly degenerates and the progesterone production is decreased. The lining of the uterus degenerates and breaks down, and menstruation begins. Menstrual flow consists of the secretions from endometrial glands, cells, blood from the broken down capillaries and the unfertilised ovum.

When the amount of progesterone in the blood falls to a critical level, the hypothalamus detects this, stimulates the anterior pituitary and FSH is secreted, thus the development of another ovarian follicle begins and the cycle starts again. This process is known as the Negative Feedback Mechanism, because it is made possible by the Hypothalamus detecting a lack of hormones and correcting the situation by recognising the deficit (refer to 7.1.3).

7.10.5 Infertility

Students should know that the following factors cause infertility:

In females:
- Blockage of fallopian tubes (often caused by pelvic inflammatory disease)
- Anatomical abnormalities e.g. backward tilting of the uterus
- Endocrine imbalances in the hormones involved in the menstrual cycle
- Low body weight or severe malnutrition
- Endometriosis, which occurs when uterus lining tissue escapes through the open ovarian end of the fallopian tube into the abdominal cavity, where it attaches to other organs and grows under the influence of the hormones of the menstrual cycle.

In men:
- Endocrine disorders
- Blockage of the vas deferens
- Failure of erection or ejaculation during sexual intercourse
- Surgical vasectomy
- Suppression of sperm formation due to exposure to ionising radiation (e.g. X-rays), chemotherapy and other drugs.
- Low sperm count or poor sperm motility.

Students should know that stress can be a major factor contributing to this and affecting both men and women. They should appreciate the effect reflexology may have in reversing infertility and that recent publicity has increased the number of prospective parents that are being referred to reflexologists to assist in this process.

In order to be able to communicate with such clients reassuringly, students should know the latest acronyms and terminology of the processes for assisted conception, such as IVF and GIFT, be aware of what is involved and the names of the medication commonly used and the extent and limitations of the part reflexology can play in this.

7.10.5 The changes that happen at birth to the baby's heart and blood vessels

Students should be able to demonstrate understanding of the changes that happen at birth to the baby's heart and pulmonary and hepatic blood vessels: They should understand that before birth, whilst oxygen is supplied from the mother via the placenta, the baby's blood bypasses the lungs via a valve-like opening in the septum of the heart between the right and left atria, and called the foramen ovale, and a further bypass in the pulmonary artery to the aorta, called the ductus arteriosus.

After birth, when pulmonary circulation is established, the pressure of blood in the left atrium is higher and the valve-like membranes close the foram ovale. The pulmonary artery by-pass then closes too. Eventually these closures become permanent due to fibrosis.

'Hole in the heart' occurs when the membranes do not close the opening in the septum, causing immediate problems for the baby if the 'hole' remains totally open or problems of poor development in early childhood if there is partial closure.

7.11 System 9 – The Nervous System

Components: Central nervous system (CNS) – Brain, spinal cord
Peripheral nervous system (PNS) – cranial and spinal nerves
Autonomic nervous system (ANS) – sympathetic and parasympathetic systems
The organs of special sense – Eyes (sight), ears (hearing and balance), nose (olfactory mechanism), tongue (taste) and sensory receptors (touch)

Students should be taught to know the Nervous System consists of two main divisions:
- The Central Nervous System
- The Peripheral Nervous System

Each student should be aware the Nervous System is one of the first systems of the body to develop. This system works with the Endocrine System to assist in the regulation of the body processes. It is responsible for interpreting information from the internal and external environment and is constantly communicating this information to the body and co-ordinating every movement both conscious and unconscious.

7.11.1 Central Nervous System

Students should know the Central Nervous System consists of the brain and the spinal cord.

They should be able to describe the human brain as a complex mass of nervous tissue that lies within the skull and each brain is a unique pattern, which is determined by both genes and experience. It requires a tremendous amount of energy and uses up to 20% of the body's oxygen and much of its glucose supply. The brain in general is soft and heavy and weighs about 1.5 kgs. It is enclosed in the skull and is cushioned by cerebrospinal fluid.

Students should be able to describe the structure and function of the components of the Brain and label on a given diagram: Cerebrum, Brainstem, Medulla Oblongata, and Cerebellum, Hypothalamus and Thalamus.

The Brain

The brain can be subdivided into three distinct, interdependent structures. Students should be aware of the following structure and functions of these three sections and be able to recall at least two facts from each.

1. Cerebrum

Outermost portion of the brain, which is divided into two halves – the left and the right cerebral hemispheres, each of which is divided into 4 lobes (temporal, frontal, parietal, occipital). This is the seat of consciousness and is the main centre for response to nerve stimulus. It deals with memory, learning, language and intelligence. About 90% of all nerve cells are in the cerebral cortex.

The folded or convoluted outer surface of the cerebrum is known as the cerebral cortex and these folds increase the surface area of the brain, allowing many more neurons to be present. The cortex is about 3mm thick. The cortex is responsible for integrating the sensory information into meaningful perceptual images and also is involved in the response mechanism. The cortex or outer layer is often referred to as grey matter as it contains the cell bodies of the neurons. The white matter is found below the cortex and contains the axons or neurons. The student should also be aware that there are various sections of the cerebrum involved with sensory, motor and association control.

Students should have worked with, and appreciate the significance to reflexology of, the motor homunculus and the sensory homunculus.

2. Brainstem

The stalk of the brain – consisting of the midbrain, the area of the brain which deals with posture and involuntary movements, and the Medulla Oblongata which controls vital centres that regulate the heart, lungs and breathing rate. The reticular formation controls sleep. Through the brainstem pass all the nerve fibres relaying signals of sensory input and efferent (response) output between the spinal cord and higher brain centres. In addition the brainstem gives rise to 10 of the 12 pairs of cranial nerves, whose axons innervates the muscles and glands of the head and many organs in the thoracic and abdominal cavities.

3. Cerebellum

Situated behind the Pons and immediately below the posterior portion of the cerebrum. It is oval in shape and has two hemispheres. This part of the brain is responsible for producing nerve signals necessary for smooth balanced and coordinated movements. This centre controls motion, motor activity and the actions of voluntary muscles.

Hypothalamus

This is involved in temperature control and contains centres for Autonomic Nervous System e.g. control of the heart, blood pressure, metabolism.

Thalamus

Relay centres for sensation. Pain is appreciated here.

The student should be aware of the anatomical positioning of the above components and be able to recognise and label each one.

Ventricles

Within the brain there are four irregular shaped spaces containing cerebrospinal fluid (CSF).

The Spinal Cord

The Spinal Cord extends from the opening at the base of the skull down to the second lumbar vertebra and is the interface between the brain and the Peripheral Nervous System. It is approximately 45cm long and has the thickness of the little finger. It is an extension of the brain stem. It is cushioned by CSF and is set within the bony vertebrae. Thirty-one pairs of spinal nerves leave the spinal cord.

The Spinal cord has the opposite set up to the brain – white matter on the outside (axons) and grey matter (cell bodies) on the inside. The spinal cord relays information about the internal/external environment to the brain. The brain then relays responses to the Peripheral Nervous System via the spinal cord.

Protection

The CNS is protected by bone, specialised membranes and a unique fluid. The student should be aware of the skull, and the three membranes, known as the meninges which work together with the cerebrospinal fluid (CSF) to protect and support the brain and nerve cells of the spinal cord. The skull provides protection on the outside.

The meninges are protective membranes which form three individual layers that wrap right round the brain and spinal cord for protection.

Dura mater, the outermost membrane layer binds tightly to the inside of the skull. Arachnoid membrane (resembling a spidery web) is the middle membrane. Pia mater, the inner membrane, attaches directly to the surface of the cerebrum. This follows the contours of the brain.

The Dura mater and arachnoid maters are separated by a potential space, the subdural space. The Arachnoid and Pia maters are separated by the subarachnoid space, containing CSF.

Cerebrospinal Fluid – This fluid is produced by specialised capillaries known as Choroid Plexuses, which line the ventricles of the brain, and bathes the entire nervous system. It consists of water, glucose, proteins, vitamins and other nutrients.

Functions of CSF

Acts as a shock absorber between the brain and the skull. Forms a protective barrier around the brain and spinal cord. Supports the structure of the Central Nervous System, by exerting a pressure. It is involved in the metabolic processes by exchanging substances between the brain and CSF.

7.11.2 Peripheral Nervous System

The Peripheral Nervous System consists of:
- 31 Pairs of Spinal Nerves
- 12 Pairs of Cranial Nerves
- Autonomic Nervous System

The Peripheral Nervous System is further subdivided:
- Afferent division (sensory) that relays information from the environment to the brain. The cell bodies are found in ganglia located beyond the brain or spinal cord.
- Efferent division (motor)
  - Somatic nervous system innervates the skeletal muscle
  - Autonomic nervous system innervates the smooth muscle, cardiac muscle or glands. It controls involuntary body functions to maintain a constant internal environment. It also regulates blood pressure and body temperature.

Nerve processes in the peripheral nervous system which transmit signals to and from the central nervous system, are grouped in bundles called nerves, whereas the individual axons are called nerve fibres. There are no nerves in the central nervous system.

Nerve fibres (axons) are wrapped in layers of a Schwann cell membrane and can either be myelinated for rapid electrical transmission or unmyelinated.

All the spinal nerves contain processes of both afferent and efferent neurons.

Afferent Nerves

The afferent nerves relay information from sensory receptors/organs about changes in the internal/external environment back via the spinal cord to the brain for interpretation.

Efferent Nerves

The efferent nerves relay a response message to the muscle, gland etc (i.e. the effector). The student would be expected to know the five main nerve plexus of the spinal nerves and the areas that they served. The student would be expected to know the 12 pairs of cranial nerves and the areas that they serve.

7.11.3 The Autonomic Nervous System

Students should be able to restate that The Autonomic Nervous System controls the involuntary functions of the body to help maintain a constant internal environment. They should know it controls the automatic activities of cardiac and smooth muscle and the activities of glands. It also plays a part in temperature control.

The Autonomic Nervous System is divided into two parts:

1. The Sympathetic Nervous System

This system prepares the body for vigorous activity (fight or flight).
Students should be able to recall some of the following effects of SNS:
- Pupils dilate, focus on distant objects
- Thick, viscous saliva production – dry mouth
- Trachea open channel maintained
- Bronchial tubes dilate
- Lung blood vessels dilate
- Increased cardiac output
- The adrenals secrete stress hormones
- Liver produces more glucose and releases it
- Kidneys decrease urine output
- Stomach decreases production of digestive enzymes
- Intestinal food movement slows down
- Bladder sphincter muscles constrict
- Blood vessels in skin constrict
- Sweat pores open, hair stands on end
- Major blood vessels to legs dilate

2. The Parasympathetic Nervous System

This system has an inhibitory effect, preparing the body for rest. It works to conservation of body energy. It works in contrast to the SNS. Students should be able to recall some of the following effects of PSN:
- Lacrimal glands produce tears
- Pupils constrict, focus on nearby objects
- Nasal glands produce mucus

- Thin copious saliva production
- Trachea and bronchial tubes constrict
- Decreased cardiac output – heart slows down
- Liver stores glucose
- Stomach increases digestive
- Pancreas secretes enzymes and insulin
- Intestinal food movement speeds up
- Bladder sphincter muscle relaxes
- Sexual organs lubricated in women, erection of penis and clitoris

Students should also be taught to recognise some of the above effects occurring during reflexology treatment and relate this to relaxation of the client. Student's attention should be drawn to the fact that this system contains the solitary reference to the solar plexus (coeliac ganglion) whereas in reflexology practice this reflex area is probably referred to and worked more than any other.

Both the Sympathetic and Parasympathetic Nervous systems work to create homeostasis within the body systems.

The student should also be aware of the role of the vagus nerve and the adrenals in the above systems.

The student should also be aware of the role of the Hypothalamus and thermoreceptors and how these communicate with the nervous system to control temperature in the body.

Neurone

The student should be able to identify the three main types of neurones and their basic structures.

A nerve is made up of a bundle of neurones or nerve cells that are enclosed in a tube of connective tissue.

A neurone or nerve cell is designed to receive stimuli and conduct impulses.

There is a space between one neurone and another called a synapse and this ensures that messages travel in one direction only. Impulses arriving at a synapse cause the release of chemicals that diffuse across the gap or space and stimulate production of impulses in the next neurone.

There are three main type of nerve cell:
- **Sensory or afferent** – receive stimuli from sensory organs and receptors in the external or internal environment and transmit the impulse to the spinal cord and brain (CNS).
- **Motor or efferent** – conduct impulses away from the brain and the CNS to muscles or glands to activate a response.
- **Associate or relay** – carries impulse from a sensory neurone through the brain and spinal cord and then passes the impulse to a motor neurone.

Nerve cell components

Students should know the Nerve Cell Component parts as: Dendrite, cell body, axon, nucleus, motor end plate, myelin sheath, Nodes of Ranvier, synapse and be able to label these on a blank diagram. They should know the structure and function of these components to be:

Dendrite

Dendrites are projections from the main cell body which collect signals from other neurons. They increase the surface area for receiving incoming signals.

Cell Body

This is the main part of the neuron. It collects information from other cells and decides what is passed on. It contains a nucleus. These are found in grey matter in the cerebral cortex and inside the spinal cord.

Axon

The axon or nerve fibre is a single process (possibly 100cm long) extending from the cell body to make connections with other neurons.

Motor end plate

The point where the nerve supply enters a muscle.

Myelin sheath

A layer of fatty insulation that speeds up transmission of nerve signals.

Nodes of Ranvier

Gaps in the myelin sheath where impulses skip from node to node.

Synapse

The space between neurones. This is where the electrical impulse from a neurone travels across via chemical neurotransmitters to the next neurone in order to trigger the second neurone to generate its own electrical impulse.

The student should also be aware of a Reflex Arc.

Properties of a Neuron
Students should be aware that the properties of a neuron are:
- Irritability – the ability to initiate nerve impulses in response to stimuli; and
- Conductivity – the ability to transmit an impulse from the brain to muscles, glands etc.

7.11.4 Functions of the Nervous System

It allows the body to respond to changes in the internal or external environment

The nervous system is responsible for the conscious experience which reflects the thinking process e.g. self awareness, reasoning, ideas, emotional feeling, concentration, imagination etc.

Any phenomena we attribute to the mind are believed to be related to the activities of the nerve cells.

Human behaviour – and internal functions of the body are regulated by the joint communication of the Nervous and Endocrine systems working together.

The cerebral cortex is associated with the thinking processes and is responsible for the initiation and control of voluntary muscle contraction.

7.11.5 The Organs of Special Sense

The main receptors

The importance to reflexology theory of understanding the functions of the main sensory receptors in the skin and other tissue and the various types of touch they respond to should be emphasised to students.

The student should be able to identify on a blank diagram the main sensory receptors in a cross section of skin: Merkel's disc, Meissner's corpuscle, Ruffini's corpuscle, Pacinian corpuscle, Krause's end bulbs, sensory receptors of the hair shaft and general free nerve endings.

In addition to the above the role of Golgi tendon organs, muscle spindles, and joint kinaesthetic receptors should be covered.

Students should be aware that the range of sensation that the above receptors detect is – light and deep pressure, deflection (hair), high and low frequency vibration, stretch, touch, heat, cold and pain.

Students should cover the following classification of receptors and know the definitions of each: chemoreceptors, mechanoreceptors, nociceptors, photoreceptors, proprioceptors and thermoreceptors.

The meaning tonic, phasic and kinaesthetic in relation to sensory reception should be known.

Skin
Structure
The student should be able to identify on a blank diagram the component parts of a cross section of skin including the epidermis (including 5 main layers), dermis, sweat glands, hair follicle, sebaceous gland, arector pili, blood vessels, subcutaneous tissue, collagen fibres, melanocytes.

Function
See The Integumentary System Section 7.3

Tongue
Structure
The student should understand the mechanism of taste and that receptor cells known as taste buds are located on the surface of the tongue, the palate, throat and epiglottis and respond to particular flavours. Taste signals are picked up from various areas of the tongue by nerve fibres from one of four cranial nerves.

Function
Students should know the functions of the tongue to be to aid mastication; to aid swallowing; to aid in identification of food taste and suitability. The role of the tongue in dental hygiene should be taught.

Nose
Structure
Components – olfactory bulb, olfactory receptor cells, olfactory epithelium, cilia and olfactory bulb.

Students should be able to identify these component parts on a diagram and be able to state the function of each.

The student should understand the mechanism of smell and be aware that more than 10,000 odours can be detected by the olfactory system.

Function

Students should know the functions of the nose to be to aid in the sense of taste; to transmit odour sensation to the brain; that recognition of odours affects the emotional response. The relationship of the nose to the respiratory processes should be repeated.

Eye

Structure

Component parts: conjunctiva, sclera, cornea, choroids, iris, pupil, lens, ciliary body, aqueous humour, vitreous humour, retina, fovea, blind spot, optic nerve, eye muscles, eyeball, eyelids, lachrymal or tear glands. Students should be able to identify these component parts on a diagram and be able to state the function of each.

The student should be aware that light stimuli are received through the eye and transmitted to the brain via the optical nerve to give us our sense of sight. The eye has three main layers known as tunics.

Function

Students should know the functions of the eye to be to transmit visual images and convert them to nerve impulses which register in the brain via the optic nerve; that the eyelids protect the eye from dirt and dust; that tears aid the cleaning of the eyes and that the eyes also aid balance.

Ear

Structure

Component parts: Pinna, Auricle, External auditory meatus, Tympanic membrane, mastoid, styloid process, auditory ossicles i.e. malleus (hammer), incus (anvil) and strapes (stirrup), oval window, cochlea, labyrinth, perilymph, auditory nerve, three semi-circular canals and Eustachian tube. Students should be able to identify these component parts on a diagram and be able to state the function of each.

The student should be aware that the ear is an organ of hearing and balance and that there are three main parts. The external ear protects and is lined with hair and glands that produce wax. It collects sound waves and conducts their vibrations towards the middle ear. The middle ear consists of auditory ossicles that transmit sound to the inner ear via a membrane and sensory hair cells. The inner ear translates vibrations into nerve messages to the brain. The three semi-circular canals control balance.

The student should also know of the Eustachian Tube and its connection with atmospheric pressure.

Function

Students should know the functions of the ear to be to transmit sound waves and convert them to nerve impulses to the brain. To aid balance dependent on impulses received.

Health

Deafness and the various reasons for this condition. Glue ear. Noise pollution and environmental factors responsible for loss of hearing.

7.12 System 10 – The Skeletal System

Components: Bone, bone marrow, synovial fluid & membrane, cartilage, ligaments

Students need to understand the skeleton is the body's framework of bones. The skeleton gives strength and support so that humans remain upright on two legs, protects underlying organs and, by the attachment of muscles, facilitates movement.

Students should know the skeleton is divided into the axial and appendicular.

7.12.1 Bones

They should be able to recall the number of bones in the skeleton and be able to label a diagram of the skeleton with the bones listed in Table 7.3. Students will be expected to label diagrams of the bones of the hand and foot in their entirety.

7.12.2 Bone marrow

They should understand the functions of bone marrow and the role it plays in the production of blood cells.

7.12.3 Cartilage and ligaments

Students should understand the tissue structure of cartilage and appreciate why it is more suitable than bone where it is used in the body. The tissue structure of ligaments should be able to be recounted and their function in attaching to bone.

7.12.4 Bone structure and composition

They must know the difference between compact and cancellous bones. An understanding of the terms 'long', 'short' 'flat', 'irregular' and 'sesamoid' is expected.

7.12.5 Joints

Students should be able to complete the table of classification of joints shown in Table 7.12.5 below and be able to include an example of each.

Table 7.12.5: Classification of joints with examples

Fixed or fibrous	Cartilaginous or semi-moveable	Synovial or freely moveable					
Examples	Synovial types	Plane/ gliding	Ball and socket	Hinge	Condyloid	Pivot	Saddle
Skull	Vertebrae	Foot	Hip	Elbow	Wrist	Atlas/axis	Hallux

Students should also be able to label the components of a typical synovial joint on a blank diagram.

7.13   System 11 – The Muscular System

Components: Muscles – Skeletal (striated), smooth and cardiac, tendons

Students should understand the principal function of the muscular system is to produce movement of the skeleton and other organs of the body with the attendant functions of maintaining posture and heat production.

7.13.1 Muscle types

Students must be able to recall:

- that there are over 600 muscles (excluding the micro-erector muscle of each hair) that make up the system and these can be divided into two categories – *voluntary* muscle which can be controlled at will and *involuntary* muscle that continues working automatically under the direction of the autonomic nervous system.

- that there are 3 types of muscle:
  1. *striated* (striped) or *skeletal muscle* which is voluntary and is attached to bones;
  2. *smooth* or *visceral, involuntary muscle* found in hollow internal organs like the bladder, blood vessels, stomach and intestines;
  3. *cardiac muscle* – the striated, involuntary muscle of the heart

Understanding of terms

Students should be aware of these characteristic terms relating to muscles: excitability, contractability, extensibility, elasticity and the antagonistic nature of muscle pairs.

Understanding of the terms origin and insertion is expected together with the ability to recognise these sites on the actual leg and foot and arm and hand.

Names of muscles

Recall of the location and name of muscles and tendons will be limited to the list in **Addenda – Table 7.3** i.e. those which the reflexologist will be more likely to need: the leg and foot, arm and hand, and those muscles more commonly damaged – neck and shoulders and back.

7.13.2 Tendons

Understanding of tendons will be limited to the type of tissue of which they are made and that they connect from bone to muscle and differ from ligaments that attach bone to bone.

ADDENDA TO SECTION 7

Examples of the tabular format of A& P:

Table 7.1: Overview of human body systems – component parts

Body system	Component body part, organ or fluid
Integumentary	Skin, hair and nails
Respiratory	Naso-pharynx, larynx, trachea, bronchi & bronchioles and lungs. Alveoli, diaphragm and intercostal muscles as sub divisions
Cardiovascular	Heart, blood, blood vessels: arteries, veins, capillaries
Lymphatic	Lymph fluid, lymph vessels, lymph nodes (organs), lymph nodules, thoracic duct, lymphatic duct, spleen, thymus and tonsils
Digestive	Mouth, teeth, tongue, salivary glands, oesophagus, cardiac sphincter, stomach, duodenum, small intestines, large intestines (colon), rectum, anus. Accessory organs: Liver, pancreas, gall bladder
Urinary	Kidneys, ureters, urinary bladder, urethra, urine
Endocrine	Pituitary gland, (with hypothalamus), pineal gland, thyroid gland, parathyroid glands, adrenal glands, pancreas (islets of Langerhans), gonads – ovaries & testes, hormones
Reproductive	Female – Breasts (mammary glands), ovaries, ova, fallopian (uterine) tubes, vagina, vulva Male – Testes, vas deferens, prostate gland, sperm, penis
Nervous	Central nervous system (CNS) – Brain, spinal cord Peripheral nervous system (PNS) – cranial and spinal nerves Autonomic nervous system (ANS) – sympathetic and parasympathetic systems The organs of special sense – Eyes (sight), ears (hearing and balance), nose (olfactory mechanism), tongue (taste) sensory receptors (touch)
Muscular	Muscles – Skeletal (striated), smooth & cardiac, tendons
Skeletal	Bone, bone marrow, synovial fluid & membrane, cartilage, ligaments

Examples of the tabular format of A& P:

Table 7.2: The respiratory system

Component	Structure	Function	Disorder
Naso-pharynx	Nose: Cartilage, 2 nostrils pointed down lined with hair (cilia), mucous secreting cells, blood vessels.	Facilitates ventilation . Nose shape safely lets air in and out. Incoming air is filtered, warmed and moistened on way to larynx	Sinusitis Rhinitis
	Pharynx: 5" long funnel of skeletal muscle, mucous lined	Passageway for air and food, resonating chamber for vocal cords and housing for tonsils	Pharyngitis
Larynx	Cartilage voice box containing vocal cords and epiglottis	To produce speech	Laryngitis
Trachea	5–8 inch flexible tube of connective tissue supported by C-shaped rings of cartilage	To protect airway as neck bends	Tracheitis
Bronchi	2 tubes, 1 to each lung, supported by cartilage, lined with ciliated membrane	Continuing warming & moistening airway Cilia move mucous and dust particles toward the pharynx to be expelled	Bronchitis COPD (chronic obstructive pulmonary disorder)
Bronchioles	The bronchi divide into increasingly smaller tubes ending as very fine ciliated bronchioles, without cartilage, in the lung substance	Delivery of air to and from alveoli	
Lungs – alveoli	2 lungs, right has 3 lobes, left only 2. Each lobe comprises numerous lobules ending in 300 million alveoli – pouches of squamous epithelial tissue	Exchange of gases to and from bloodstream	Asthma Cancer Pneumonia
Pleural membranes and cavity	Serous membrane lining the thoracic cavity and covering each lung with potential space containing serous fluid	Pleura provides protection and facilitates smooth gliding during expansion and recoil of lungs	Emphysema Pleurisy Pneumathorax
Diaphragm	Dome-shaped skeletal muscle forming floor of thoracic cavity	Diaphragm contraction increases vertical dimension of thoracic cavity drawing air into lungs	Hiccoughs
Intercostal muscles	2 sets of skeletal muscle, internal & external	Allows movement of ribs to increase and decrease size of thoracic cavity	

Table 7.3: Specific body parts that require Recall to label diagrams

Body part	Blood vessels	Bones	Muscles	Tendons	Nerves
Legs/Feet	Iliac artery Femoral artery Popliteal artery Ant.Tibial artery Post.Tibial artery Plantar arch Digital arteries	Femur Tibia Fibula Tarsals Metatarsals Phalanges	Quadriceps & Hamstrings Tibialis anterior Gastrocnemious Soleus Peroneus longus Retinaculum Hallucis longus flexor Extensor Digitorum longus Gluteus	Achilles Flexor hallucis longus	Sciatic Femoral Gluteal Tibial Peroneal Saphenous Plantar
Arms/ Hands	Brachial artery Radial artery Ulnar artery Palmar arch Digital arteries	Humerus Radius Ulna Carpals Metacarpals Phalanges	Triceps Biceps Extensor Digitorum Flexor and extensor Carpi Ulnaris Flexor and abductor Pollicis brevis Flexor Digitorum superficialis	Flexor digitorum profundus	Radial Medial Subscapular Brachial Cranial
General Thorax	Ascending aorta Innominate artery Subclavial artery Carotoid arteries Coronary arteries Jugular vein	Clavicle Ribs	Pectorals Latissimus Dorsi Intercostals Rectus Abdominus Erectus Spinae Trapezius		Phrenic Intercostal Cervical Pectoral Cranial
Abdomen	Hepatic artery Hepatic portal vein Mesenteric artery Femoral artery Splenic artery Iliac artery Descending Aorta Renal arteries	Pelvis Sacro/iliac	Internal Obliques External Obliques Rectus Abdominus		Phrenic Cervical Femoral Sciatic
Spine Plexus Nerves	Intercostal arteries	Vertebrae: 7 Cervical 12 Thoracic 5 Lumbar 5 Sacral 4 Coccyx	Sterno mastoid Intercostals Sacro spinalis		Brachial Plexus Lumbar Plexus Sacral Plexus Coeliac (Solar) 12 Cranial

Table 7.4: Anatomical Regional Terms – to be labelled on a blank diagram

	Term	Location		Term	Location
1	Abdominal	Trunk below diaphragm	21	Leg	Lower limb esp. knee – foot
2	Arm	Upper limb, shoulder – elbow	22	Lumbar	Loin, lower back & side rib-pelvis
3	Axillary	Armpit area			
4	Brachial	Arm	23	Mammary	Breasts
5	Buccal	Inner surface of cheek	24	Occipital	Back of head
6	Calcaneal	Heel of foot	25	Opthalmic	Eyes
7	Carpal	Wrist	26	Oral	Mouth
8	Celiac(celiac)	Abdomen	27	Orbital	Bony cavity containing eyeball
9	Cephalic	Head	28	Palmar	Palm of hand
10	Cervical	Neck region	29	Patellar	Knee
11	Costal	Ribs	30	Pectoral	Chest
12	Cranial	Skull	31	Pedal	Foot
13	Cubital	Elbow or forearm	32	Pelvic	Bony ring girdling lower trunk
14	Cutaneous	Skin	33	Perineal	Area from anus to pubic arch
15	Femoral	Thigh: Lower limb, hip-knee	34	Plantar	Sole of the foot
16	Forearm	Upper limb, elbow-wrist	35	Popliteal	Area behind the knee
17	Frontal	Forehead	36	Sacral	Base of spine
18	Gluteal	Buttocks	37	Tarsal	Ankle
19	Groin	Depressed area between abdomen and thigh	38	Thoracic	Chest, trunk between neck and diaphragm
20	Inguinal	Groin	39	Umbilical	Navel, site of umbilical cord entry

Table 7.5: Anatomical Directional Terms – to be labelled on a blank diagram

	Term	Meaning/location
1	Superior	Toward the head /upper part
2	Inferior or (caudad)	Toward the feet/lower part (toward the tail)
3	Anterior (ventral)	Front surface
4	Posterior (dorsal)	Rear surface (behind), back
5	Medial	Closer to the midline of body
6	Lateral	Toward one side of the body
7	Proximal (especially limbs)	Closer to the midline
8	Distal (especially limbs)	Farther from the midline
9	Superficial	Toward the surface of body
10	Deep	Away from body surface
11	Parietal	Forming wall of body cavity
12	Visceral	Pertaining to an internal organ
13	Ipsilateral	On the same side of the body
14	Contralateral	On opposite side of body

Body Planes

15	Sagittal	Divides into right and left
16	Transverse	Divides superior and inferior
17	Frontal (coronal)	Divides anterior and posterior – front and back

Anatomy & Physiology

8 RELATING REFLEXOLOGY TO HEALTH

Recommended Teacher Contact Hours – **10**	Expected Home Study Hours – **100**

This section is essential to the concept of reflexology as a *medical treatment,* as it was first intended. (Ingham, 1938)

This distinction is emphasised in the light of awards that may cater for students who intend to work in the health and beauty sector, working from salons, gyms and home. Some argue that there is no such distinction and that reflexology is universal and at a single level in all sectors including health. Whilst this ideal has not yet been achieved, the application of the National Occupational Standards and this Curriculum by training providers and awarding bodies will work toward a single level at which all reflexologists will work as clinical practitioners.

8.1 List of Diseases and Disorders

This list of over 100 conditions has been drawn from the experience of clinically-oriented reflexologists, some having over 25 years of practical experience, as being those conditions most likely to be encountered in the course of running a practice. Such a list could never be exhaustive, but is wide enough to equip a student to work with autonomy as a practitioner. They should have the understanding and self assurance to decide whether to treat or refer and how to adapt treatment to each client with their health problem.

8.1.1 Nail and foot disorders

The list includes a section of foot disorders along with a section for disorders of the nail (both hand and foot), invaluable as a diagnostic tool. This will help to recognise contraindicated feet, occasions on which to refer and pointers to other related disorders that may not be immediately obvious.

Much consideration has been given to whether this list should be related to, or an integral part of, the various systems in the A & P section. However, the inclusion of an alphabetical presentation of the list has been chosen with the rationale that the workbooks produced to facilitate training for this section will be useful as a self-produced alphabetical reference book to which each student can refer.

LEARNING OUTCOMES FROM SECTION 8

After completing this section of the curriculum a student will be able to:

Tab 8A   *Demonstrate* an awareness of over 100 (one hundred) disorders commonly encountered by reflexologists, *recall* the conventional treatment/medication prescribed, *describe* the condition and *state* its symptoms. As a result of this information *analyse* the disorder in relation to the reflexes likely to be disordered and *synthesise* a treatment plan, *evaluating* whether the treatment will need adapting to the particular client presenting.

LEARNING OUTCOMES MAPPED AGAINST ASSESSMENT TOOLS
(See Appendix 2)

Tool	Learning Outcome Verbs
Case Studies	demonstrate awareness, describe, evaluate, recall, state, synthesise
Client Studies	demonstrate awareness, describe, evaluate, recall, state, synthesise
Home Treatments	demonstrate awareness
Blank Feet/Hand Diagrams to locate Reflex Points/Areas	
Blank Diagrams of Body Parts to Labels A&P Items	
2000 to 5000-word Assignments	
At level 2	analyse, demonstrate awareness, describe, evaluate, recall, state
At level 3	analyse, demonstrate awareness, evaluate, recall, state, synthesise
Interim (Formative) Assessments (Written)	demonstrate awareness, describe, recall, state
Interim (Formative) Assessments (Practical)	demonstrate awareness, describe, recall, state
Final (Summative) Assessments (Written)	analyse, demonstrate awareness, describe, evaluate, recall, state, synthesise
Final (Summative) Assessments (Practical)	analyse, demonstrate awareness, describe, evaluate, recall, state, synthesise
Professional Portfolio	analyse, demonstrate awareness, evaluate, state, synthesise
Interview	demonstrate awareness, describe, evaluate, recall, state, synthesise
Project: Research based or audit	analyse, demonstrate awareness, evaluate, synthesise

Table 8A: List of diseases and disorders for consideration during the course – Related to Systems

Integumentary System
Boil
Cyst
Dermatitis
Eczema
Hyperhidrosis
Shingles (Herpes Zoster)
Wart

Respiratory System
Asthma
Bronchitis
Embolism (inc. Pulmonary)
Emphysema
Hay Fever
Hyperventilation
Pleurisy
Pneumonia
Sinusitis
Snoring
Sore throat
Whooping Cough (Pertussis)

Cardiovascular System
Anaemia
Angina
Arteriosclerosis
Atheroma
Gangrene
Heart Attack
Heart, Hole in Heart, Pacemaker fitted
Hypertension
Hypotension
Nosebleeds (Epistaxis)
Palpitations/Panic attack
Phlebitis
Raynaud's Disease Thrombosis – DVT
Varicose Ulcer
Varicose Veins

Lymphatic System
Allergies
Breast (lump in)
Cancer
Fever
HIV (and AIDS)
Influenza
Lymphoma
Lymphoedema
Mastitis
MyalgicEncephalomyelitis (ME)
Melanoma
Oedema
Thrush (Candidiasis)
Tuberculosis (TB)
Tumours

Digestive System
Cirrhosis of the liver
Crohn's Disease
Colitis (including Ulcerative Colitis)
Constipation
Diarrhoea
Diverticulitis
Flatulence
Gall Bladder, inflamed
    Gall stone

Gastroenteritis
Haemorrhoids
Hepatitis
Hiatal Hernia
Indigestion (Dyspepsia)
Irritable Bowel Syndrome (IBS)
Jaundice
Pernicious Anaemia
Spastic colon
Tooth disorders
Ulcer – apthous, duodenal, gastric, peptic

Urinary System
Cystitis
Incontinence
Nephritis
Renal Colic
Urethritis

Endocrine System
Adrenal Problems:
    Addison's disease
    Cushing's syndrome
Diabetes Insipidus
Diabetes Mellitus
Seasonal Affective Disorder (SAD)
Thyroid problems:
    Goitre
    Hyper (Thyrotoxicosis)
    Hypo (Myxoedema)

Reproductive System
Endometriosis
Fibroid
Hysterectomy
Impotence and Frigidity Infertility
Menstrual problems:
    Amenorrhoea
    Dysmenorrhoea
    Menorrhagia
    Pre-menstrual Syndrome
Post-natal Depression
Prostate Disorder

Nervous System
Alzheimer's Disease
Bell's Palsy
Depression
Ear Problems:
    Deafness
    Earache
    Glue Ear
    Tinnitus
    Vertigo
Epilepsy
Eye Problems:
Cataract
Corneal ulcer
Glaucoma
Fainting
Headache
Insomnia
Meningitis
Migraine
Motor Neurone disease
Multiple Sclerosis (MS)
Muscular Dystrophy

Neuralgia
Pain and Referred Pain
Paralysis
Parkinsons disease
Sciatica
Stress – Tension
Stroke – CVA

Skeletal System
Arthritis
Osteo
Rheumatoid
Bursitis
Frozen Shoulder
Ganglion
Golfer's Elbow
Gout
Housemaid's Knee
Osteogenesis
    Imperfecta
Osteomalacia
Osteoporosis
Spinal Disorders:
    Kyphosis
    Lordosis
    Scoliosis
PID – Prolapsed Intervertebral
    (Slipped) Disc
Synovitis
Tennis Elbow
Tendonitis
Whiplash

Muscular System
Cramp
Poliomyelitis
Rheumatism
Tetanus (Lockjaw)

Foot Disorders
Athlete's Foot
Bone Spur
Bunion (Hallux Valgus)
Callus
Chilblain
Clubbed Foot
Corn (Heloma)
Fissure (Heel)
Flat Feet (PesPlanus)
Foot Drop
Hammer Toe
High Arch (Pes Cavus)
Verruca

Nail Disorders *(including)*
Blue Nails
Discoloured Nails
Habit Tic
Ingrowing Nail
Pitting
Ridged Nails
Vertical Streaks
Koilonychia
Onychogryphosis
Onychomycosis
Onycholysis
Paronychia

Table 8B: Alphabetical list of diseases and disorders for consideration during the course

Allergies
Alzheimer's Disease
Anaemia
  Pernicious Anaemia
Angina
Arteriosclerosis
Arthritis, Osteo
Arthritis, Rheumatoid
Asthma
Atheroma

Bell's Palsy
Boil
Breast (lump in)
Bronchitis
Bursitis

Cancer
Cataract
Crohn's Disease
Colitis (inc. Ulcerative Colitis)
Constipation
Cramp
Cystitis
Cyst

Deafness
Depression
Diabetes Insipidus
Diabetes Mellitus
Diarrhoea
Diverticulitis

Earache
Eczema
Embolism (inc Pulmonary)
Emphysema
Endometriosis
Epilepsy

Fainting
Fever
Fibroid
Flatulence
Foot Disorders
  Athlete's Foot
  Bone Spur
  Bunion (Hallux Valgus)
  Callus
  Chilblain
  Clubbed Foot
  Corn (Heloma)
  Fissure (Heel)
  Flat feet (Pes planus)

Foot Drop
Hammer Toe
High Arch (Pes cavus)
  Verruca
Frozen Shoulder

Gall Bladder *Inflamed/ stone*
Ganglion
Gangrene
Gastroenteritis
Glaucoma
Glue Ear
Golfer's Elbow
Gout

Hay Fever
Headache
HIV (and AIDS)
Heart Attack
Heart, Hole in
Heart, Pacemaker fitted
Haemorrhoids
Hiatal Hernia
Housemaid's Knee
Hyperhidrosis
*Hyper*tension
*Hypo*tension
Hyperventilation
Hysterectomy

Impotence, and Frigidity
Incontinence
Indigestion (Dyspepsia)
Infertility
Influenza
IBS – *Irritable Bowel Syndrome*
Insomnia

Kidney Disorders:
  Nephritis
  Renal Colic
  Urethritis

Liver Disorders
  Cirrhosis
  Hepatitis
  Jaundice
Lymphoma
Lymphoedema

Mastitis
ME
  Myalgicencephalo- myelitis

Melanoma
Meningitis
Menstrual
  Amenorrhoea
  Dysmenorrhoea
  Menorrhagia
Migraine
MND
  Motor neurone disease
MS
  Multiple sclerosis
MD
  Muscular Dystrophy

Nail Disorders:
  Blue Nails
  Discoloured Nails
  Habit Tic
  Ingrowing Nail
  Pitting
  Ridged Nails
  Vertical Streaks
  Koilonychia
  Onychogryphosis
  Onychomycosis
  Onycholysis
  Paronychia
Neuralgia
Nosebleeds (Epistaxis)

Osteogenesis Imperfecta
Osteomalacia
Osteoporosis
Oedema

Pain & Referred Pain
Palpitations/Panic attack
Paralysis
Parkinson's disease
Phlebitis
Pleurisy
Pre-menstrual Syndrome
Pneumonia
Poliomyelitis
Post Natal Depression
Prostate Disorder
Psoriasis

Raynaud's Disease
Rheumatism

SAD *Seasonal Affective Disorder*

Sciatica
Shingles *Herpes Zoster*
Sinusitis
Skin disorders
  Dermatitis
  Prickly Heat
  Scabies
Snoring
Sore throat
Spastic Colon
Spinal
  Kyphosis
  Lordosis
  Scoliosis
  Cervical
  Thoracic
  Lumbar
  Sacrum
  PID (*Slipped Disc*)
Stress
  Tension
Stroke
  CVA
Synovitis

Tennis Elbow
Tetanus
  Lockjaw
Tendonitis
Thrombosis
  DVT
Thrush (Candidiasis)
Thyroid
  Goitre
  Hyper (Thyrotoxicosis)
  Hypo (Myxoedema)
Tinnitus
Tooth disorders
TB (Tuberculosis)
Tumours

Ulcer
  Apthous
  Corneal
  Duodenal
  Gastric
  Peptic
  Varicose

Varicose Veins
Vertigo

Wart
Whiplash
Whooping Cough (Pertussis)

8.2 Sample from course workbook

Below is reproduced the instruction page from a course workbook of the type that the student would complete from using *biology textbooks, a medical dictionary and a BNF*. The 172 disorders can be completed in any sequence. Course hours allow 10 classroom and 100 home study and can run into year 2 (see section A1.3 in Appendix 1).

The first column of the table lists the disorder, sometimes using both its common name and its medical label. Some rows contain multiple areas – the spinal disorders, for example, include several postural problems – also a section to consider how you would approach problems of the four main areas of the spine.

The second column asks for a description of the particular disorder. Keep this brief using concise phrases rather than long sentences.

The third column is for you to list the usual symptoms with which people who suffer from this disorder commonly present. This may be completed using single words such as 'insomnia' rather than 'the client finds it hard to get off to sleep or keeps waking up'.

The fourth column is for you to enter the conventional/allopathic treatment usually given for this disorder. This may be medicine taken orally, injected or applied topically. It could be a surgical intervention, a physical treatment such as physiotherapy, psychotherapy or counselling. It may be appropriate to include investigations prior to and during treatment such as scans, blood tests, x-rays etc. An awareness of what your client is experiencing, such as the actual names of drugs and tests, can be reassuring and will help them have confidence in you and your training.

The fifth column is for you to name the areas of reflexology emphasis for that disorder. This section should list only the *primary areas* involved, as it is easy to get carried away and end up naming every reflex area that exists! This selective emphasis illustrates the integration of the body and the holistic nature of reflexology. As a guide each problem would have about *three* to *five* areas of emphasis only. If you include more areas than 3–5 the concept of emphasis becomes less relevant and is so much harder to remember. *(Compare the concise nature of Kunz & Kunz with Laura Norman's extensive listings. Remember, the entire pair of feet [or hands] is worked during a treatment anyway!)*

The sixth column, *'reasons'*, is for you to explain how and why that particular area relates to the disorder. The secret to making this workbook an effective learning aid and a future reference work is – simplicity. Keep your reasons short and repetitive using single words or short phrases only. For example, in Asthma, the Adrenal Glands are worked to emphasise their use as a Broncho-dilator; the Chest & Lung area quite simply because it is the Area Affected by this disorder and so on. The expression *'Area Affected'* or *'Area Involved'* will most likely occur in every problem on the list.

The seventh, and final*, column, 'adaptations'* is for special instructions that may apply for some conditions. For example, it would be good to write down that for Gout, if it is presenting in its common Hallux (BigToe) position, the referral area should be worked – the corresponding Thumb. Also include a reminder to start a regime of initially judicious toe rotation to gently loosen and detoxify the joint. This will be able to progress to firmer and wider rotations as the client's pain diminishes. For Verruca, note down the treatment and hygiene procedure of covering it with a plaster.

Try to *line up* the areas with the other columns so they can be easily referenced later when using this book with your clients. Use either a *straight edge* or even *different colour ink* for each line. Highlighter pens are good for this and are now available in more than 5 colours. Note the example below.

We know that you will not only find this exercise challenging and stimulating but a rewarding and essential guide for the future.

Example of Concise Workbook Layout

	Disorder	Description of Disorder	Symptoms	Reasons		Areas of Emphasis	Reasons	Adaptation?
6	Asthma	Chronic condition making exhalation difficult due to spasm in the bronchi/lungs. Attacks provoked by allergy, infection, and stress. Usually treated by bronchodilators to relax spasm and steroids to reduce bronchial inflammation	Difficulty in breathing, especially exhaling Wheezing Coughing Excess of mucus	Daily/chronic use – steroid inhaler (Brown) When needed/Acute attack – Bronchodilator Inhaler (Blue) Nebuliser	6	Chest/Lungs Area Adrenal Glands Solar Plexus (Coeliac Ganglion)	Area affected/ involved Acts as a bronchodilator Stress – is both a cause and an effect	Minimal or NIL use of powder/talc Keep hand over container top when putting down – even sight of dust can cause asthmatic distress

APPENDIX 1 COURSE

A1.1 Course Title

The name of the course will be:

Practitioner Course in Reflexology

The rationale for this being:

Practitioner: On January 30th 2003, the Prince of Wales's Foundation for Integrated Health hosted a meeting conducted by Skills for Health and attended by representatives from the Awarding Bodies, QCA and representatives from the Massage, Aromatherapy and Reflexology professional organisations discuss the Role of the Practitioner. At that meeting it was proposed that the title **Reflexology Therapist** could refer to:

'An individual who has been trained to use conventional reflexology techniques as directed by their manager, clinical supervisor or the clients' GP, or they may run their own reflexology practice within the health and beauty sector.

The therapist will be trained to recognise/identify a comprehensive set of contra-indications, many of which will necessitate obtaining the approval of the client's doctor before treatment. The therapist's insurance will usually reflect the need for a doctor's written approval before treatment.'

Whereas a **Reflexology Practitioner** could refer to:

'An individual who has been trained and educated to autonomously manage their own practice to assess and treat clients using conventional reflexology techniques. This would usually be without the need to obtain consent from the client's doctor and would involve the recognition/identification of a comprehensive set of contra-indications.

The general public should be in a position to make an informed choice about whom they should seek treatment from. Members of the public should be able to seek out a reflexology practitioner when they require treatment for a (previously diagnosed) clinical or medical condition equally they should be able to seek out a reflexology therapist when they need a stress relieving treatment.'

(FIH Document 28th March 2003)

It is the feeling of the Education and Training Working Group that this curriculum would prepare a reflexologist to practice at the level of autonomy and skill that matches the definition of a Practitioner, and it will be appropriate for this to be reflected in the title.

The term 'Clinical'

This term was originally included in the title to indicate that the practitioner has received training that enables him/her to:

- apply safe and effective reflexology techniques to a broad range of clients and
- adapt these treatments to a wide range of clinical conditions with which clients may present.

As a result of valuable feedback from the first draft, the 'EaT' group discussed the concept that *all* Reflexology treatments should be 'clinical' and that it may be appropriate to discontinue the use of this word.

This discussion was also fuelled by the current conflicting uses of this term: At least one organisation uses the term 'Clinical' to refer to *the environment* where the therapist/practitioner works, namely a *clinic* or within the *healthcare environment*. Others use 'Clinical' to refer to the **training and ability** to work with clinical (medical, health) problems or situations.

When this curriculum is used nationally there should be no need for any practitioner to feel they need to use additional terms to indicate they operate at a different level to a 'well-being' therapist. This minimum curriculum is intended to produce practitioners who can work with clinical conditions. The intention is that the public can be assured that once the curriculum is in place to receive the designation 'reflexologist' will denote a practitioner who is trained to work equally as well with people who seek help with clinical conditions and those who desire a relaxing treatment.

In anticipation of the national use of the Core Curriculum/National Occupational Standards in determining the minimum requirement to become a reflexologist, the name of this training will be 'Practitioner Course in Reflexology'.

A1.2 Sector

The sector where the curriculum will be represented will be:

Health

under the designation 'Complementary Medicine' (Training Representation currently via 'Skills for Health')

A1.3 Course Hours and Duration

A1.3.1 Number of Course/Training Hours

The need to reassess of the hours and duration of the delivery of this core curriculum is closely tied with the proposed Levels of both **Training** (Vocational, or NVQ Level) and **Education** (Academic Level). It is also directly related to three other factors:

- Current Reflexology training and education provision tends to be short
- Feedback from many newly qualified 'reflexologists' is that many do not feel ready to treat 'real' clients – thus the need for a longer provision of learning and a more rigorous assessment process
- The current training requirement accepted for other complementary and conventional therapies in comparison to which reflexology should not be considered inferior

The initial review of reflexology training current in the UK at 2001/2 (see Section 1, Introduction) revealed a disparity of provision ranging from two years' duration down to two days, both extremes offering a 'diploma in reflexology'. The investigation also unearthed courses via correspondence that had no requirement to attend a training centre, no direct teacher contact or any assessment. This situation obviously cannot be tolerated and the national use of this core curriculum will substantially unify what previously has been a 'disparate profession.' (Mills and Budd, 2000)

More important, is the effect this curriculum will have upon the public as users of Reflexology. Whilst being generally safe and non-invasive with regard to physical technique, the public can be at risk from flawed hygiene procedure, ignorance of contraindications and cautions, extremes of pressure and the non-adherence to a code of conduct and ethics. A curriculum that has little provision for these areas of practice can pose a danger to the public. Perhaps the greatest potential for harm relates to what poorly-trained reflexologists *may say to clients/patients* with regard to promises of cure, exaggerated claims, the 'diagnosing' of non-existent disease, the ignoring of significant symptoms or unnecessary requests for GP's permission to treat. A substantial training period can eliminate these practices. Tutors will have more time to educate students effectively and time will allow those who are inclined to say the wrong things to reveal themselves, to be retrained or removed.

Since 2002 the proposal of the Reflexology Forum Education and Training group has consistently been that to satisfactorily cover the entire content of this curriculum there would need to be:

- **Recommended Teacher Contact Hours/'Guided Learning Hours': 180**
- **Anticipated Home Study Hours: 600**

Table A1.3 below provides a grid of the likely allocation of hours to the various sections of the curriculum. This will aid the process of APL and the planning of course delivery.

The assessment processes are to be included in the teacher contact hours.

Table A1.3: Allocation of Course Hours

	Section	Notes	Teacher contact hours total	Home study hours total
4	Theory	A	30	100
5	Technique	B	50	50
6	Clinical Practice	C	40	80
App 3	Client/Case Studies/External Treatment Practice	D		120
7	Anatomy & Physiology	E	50	150
8	Relating Reflexology to Heath	F	10	100
Total		**G**	**180**	**600**

Notes:

A –The higher home study hours includes the research element, which is student-led work

B – Technique is practical work so ratio of contact hours to home study is 1 to 1. In total ratio is 3.5 to 1

C – Clinical Practice requires less home study – 2 to 1

D – Case Studies and External treatment practice completely home based – no teacher hours (except assessment)

E – A & P is 3 to 1 – subject requires more self-directed study

F – R.R. to Health (Pathology) is heavily self-directed, 10 to 1, once shown the student completes the workbook

G – The total hours reflect that the bulk of teaching is in one year, leaving any more allocated time for supervised consolidation of learning with teacher support. Training providers who have concerns about cost should consider CPD or supervised practice – schemes which create income and jobs.

A1.3.2 Likely Duration of Course/Training

A Minimum of One Academic Year

The rationale for this duration is:

- to allow time for the assimilation of the course content and development of technical skill
- to enable the student to become confident as a practitioner
- to allow time for the research related project to complete or mature
- to promote public and professional perception of reflexology as a serious subject that can be perceived as Healthcare rather than 'Well being' (Many other complementary disciplines require substantially longer periods of training and command higher training and treatment costs – reflexology has been considered by some to be 'lightweight' in comparison).
- to allow the student sufficient time to perform the required number of home treatments (100) and produce the case studies (40) that need to be analysed and then written up either individually or as an assignment (see section A1.6 in this Appendix)
- A two-year duration is already established as a precedent (Appendix 8).

Academic Courses
Many universities now offer two reflexology modules in two years at academic levels 2 and 3

Vocational Training
Though the duration is not always specified by the awarding body some Vocational training providers run a two-year programme

Private Sector
The initial EaT report on reflexology education and training in the UK (see page 2) revealed many private providers run programmes significantly longer than one year

A1.4 Student Entry Requirements

A1.4 Course/Training Entry Requirements

The overriding principle for entry into reflexology training is to be inclusive without lowering standards.

Historically, those enrolling for reflexology training have been mature people, predominantly female, who have either personally benefited from reflexology or have witnessed its capacity to heal. Others have seen it as a career change, many of these being from the nursing and midwifery profession, or wish to add another dimension to their career in complementary medicine. As training becomes more structured and added to the National Framework of Qualifications, the potential for younger people to use reflexology as a first choice for a career increases, so the curriculum needs to reflect this change. The proposal of the Reflexology Forum Education and Training group is described overleaf.

Course/Training Entry Requirements

1. **Over 18 years of age upon commencement of training**
   The entry route for younger students and previous reflexology training can be seen in Appendix 6

2. **Dextrous**
   The rationale for the word 'dextrous' is that adaptation of training should be as *inclusive* as possible. Adapted techniques have been successfully learned for students with restricted manual use due to, for example, Polio. Unsighted (blind) reflexologists can be excellent, even gifted, practitioners.

   Training providers should seek to deliver adapted training for as many physical and learning difficulties as they can handle or seek to direct such prospective students to a provider who is adequately equipped. However, it has to be acknowledged that there *will be situations* when physical and/or learning difficulties preclude an individual from becoming a reflexology practitioner.

3. **Adequate command of written and spoken English**
   As verbal and written communication with clients, their carers, other health professionals and the general public are all vital to a practitioner of reflexology this entry requirement is mandatory. In addition, the course content and assessment structure requires written assignments equating to academic level 2, and students should be comfortable with providing work reflecting that level. The provision of Key Skills applies here. *(Until the resources for translation into, and training in, the Welsh language have been researched and ascertained, this UK core curriculum is in English only.)*

4. **The personal and financial resources to complete the duration of the course**
   The collective vast experience of the Reflexology Forum Education and Training group moves it to stress the importance of adequate *pre-enrolment interviews* to ensure candidates are aware of the level of academic, financial and time commitment this curriculum demands from the student. *It is important that the primary tutor conducts, or is included in these interviews.*

   At present, the responsibility for making decisions on entry requirements, particularly 2 and 3 above, lies with the tutor, who has to adapt to any special circumstances. The tutor is responsible to the training provider who has to make provision for such adaptation. If a candidate feels that an entry refusal is unfair they should follow the appeals procedure that should be readily available from the training provider via the tutor.

A1.5 First Aid Requirement

A practitioner in reflexology should hold a current First Aid Certificate
The proposal of the Reflexology Forum Education and Training group is that the award of Practitioner in Reflexology is dependent upon the student holding a current and appropriate First Aid certificate issued by a recognised body such as the British Red Cross or the St. John Ambulance.

Such certificates usually remain valid for three years after which an update is required. Students may commence practitioner training with a valid certificate or obtain one during the course. Awarding bodies should have evidence of First Aid certification before releasing a practitioner award.

A proposal of the Reflexology Forum Education and Training group is to negotiate with a leading training provider for a specific package of First Aid measures and interventions for situations that are more likely to be encountered when practicing reflexology . This will ensure that the First Aid input will reflect the consistent UK level of training and education that this curriculum along with the National Occupational Standards seeks to deliver.

A1.5.1 First Aid for Reflexologists Package

Relevant composites of a First Aid Package for Reflexologists could be:

Subjects

Making an initial assessment
Making a diagnosis
Resuscitation
Specific disorders
Emergency childbirth
Handling and transport

Specific Emergencies

The recovery position
Breathe for the casualty
Commence CPR
Abdominal pain
Allergic reactions
Asthma attack
Back injury
Choking – adult; child; baby
Convulsions – adult; child
Earache
Eye injury
Fever
Heart attack
Head injury
Hiccups
Hysteria
Shock
Sore throat
Toothache
Unconsciousness
Vomiting and diarrhoea

A1.6 Course Teacher Qualifications

The Reflexology Forum Education and Training group repeatedly came across the following criticism during the information gathering stage of the preparation of this curriculum. Tutors on reflexology courses were often not able to answer questions about clinical practice and were loath to demonstrate practical skills or instil confidence in their students. This was always due to the fact that they were not really reflexologists themselves, or teaching had taken over where practice stopped.

To put in place a Quality Assurance mechanism the proposal of the Reflexology Forum Education and Training group is that a reflexology qualification and current, ongoing experience is as important as a teaching qualification:

- **Unsupervised course tutors/course leaders** should have, in addition to their teaching qualification, or qualification in progress, **either five years** or **1000 hours continuous** and **current experience** as a **reflexology practitioner** and belong to a member organisation of the **Reflexology Forum**
- **Supervised course tutors/facilitators** should have, in addition to their teaching qualification, or qualification in progress, **either three years** or **600 hours continuous** and **current experience** as a **reflexology practitioner** and belong to a member organisation of the **Reflexology Forum**
- **The Teaching Qualification** should be a recognised award such as City and Guilds 7407 (or 7307) Stages 1 and 2, a Certificate in Education, Stage 2 or PGCE. (The Reflexology Forum Education and Training group will be compiling a list of equivalent or higher teaching qualifications to measure the suitability of applicants for teaching posts who may hold different qualifications or who may have qualified in another country and wish to teach the UK core curriculum.)
- **The Assessors Qualification** for Tutor/Assessors on competence based, vocational training is
  - A1: 'Assess candidates using a range of methods'
  - A2: 'Assess candidates' performance through observation' (those holding D32 and D33 will probably not need to reapply).
- **The Verifier** units D34 and D35 have now been replaced by:
  - V1: 'Conduct internal quality assurance of the assessment process'
  - V2: 'Conduct external quality assurance of the assessment process'

'Skills for Health' have produced guidelines for assessment and quality control of Complementary Medicine (see Appendix 7)

It is not to be interpreted that with immediate effect all teachers of reflexology currently in place must cease if they do not meet the above criteria. This would neither be practical nor desirable. From September 2006 NEW applicants who wish to teach reflexology should ensure they can evidence, or have the training underway in order that they will be able to evidence, that they have these qualifications. Existing teachers must be able to be guided by their professional organisations until the regulatory body for reflexology is able to advise.

This 'Grand parenting' principle is in use across all CAM disciplines to ensure the smooth implementation of higher standards.

APPENDIX 2 — ASSESSMENT

A2.1 Assessment Strategy

The proposal of the Reflexology Forum Education and Training group is that the assessment strategy for this reflexology core curriculum should take account of the theoretical and practical aspects of reflexology.

It will establish that the students have demonstrated a progression through the different levels of complexity by showing:
- Competence in the integration of theory and practice
- Ability to analyse, synthesise, evaluate and integrate the contribution of the different subject areas within the course to an understanding of specific topics in reflexology theory, technique, clinical practice, human biology and pathology
- An ability to integrate learning outcomes into clinical practice

Or
- An ability to demonstrate competence against a set of performance criteria relating to a broad scope of work activities and in a wide range of contexts
- To provide feedback to students in their own personal and professional development

A2.2 Assessment Scheme

The proposal of the Reflexology Forum Education and Training group is:

1. **The assessment process for practical skills should be one of Continuous Assessment**. The continuous assessor will usually be the tutor and is ideally placed to continually assess and guide the student from 'novice to expert'.
2. **The use of phase tests to continually assess theoretical skills should be encouraged.**
3. **There should be an examination/written assessment at the end of the course for which a pass mark should be achieved (or each academic year if a two-year programme).**
4. **There should also be at least one practical summative assessment at the end of the course for which a pass mark should be achieved (or each academic year if a two-year programme).** The assessor will observe a complete treatment on a genuine (unsimulated) client including consultation, full treatment, final evaluation, rebooking and treatment recording. If the pass mark (or 100% competence in the case of vocational training) is not achieved this event shall be repeatable at the discretion of assessor (and/or verifier).
5. **Regular tutorial appointments and the production of a portfolio are to be an integral part of the assessment process. This Portfolio will be a 'living document' to be continued through training assessment and into post-graduate education and will provide the basis for Continuing Professional Development (CPD).** The keeping of a personal reflective journal/diary is suggested.

Please refer to **Appendix 4** for Assessment Documentation, and Guidelines on Quality Control

A2.3 Suitable Assessment Tools

The following are suitable tools to facilitate assessment of learning outcomes:

Case Studies	A Case Study is defined as *'a course of Reflexology treatment performed outside contact hours/clinic sessions where **the tutor will not be there** to observe the practical skills of the student directly'*. **(A2.5.2)**
Client Studies	A Client Study is defined as *'a course of Reflexology treatment performed on a client during contact hours/clinic sessions **when the tutor is present** to assess the practical techniques being used by the student'*. **(A2.5.1)**
Home Treatments (or External Treatment Practice)	Refers to *'all other correctly researched, performed, evaluated and recorded treatments that are not Client Studies or Case Studies'*. **(A2.5.3)**
Blank Feet/Hand Diagrams to locate Reflex Points/Areas	Unlabelled foot or hand maps/charts that require the identification of specific reflex points/areas. Blank foot or hand outlines that require the identification and insertion of given specific reflex points/areas.

Blank Diagrams of Body Parts to Label A&P Items
2000 to 5000-word Assignments
Interim (Formative) Assessments (Written and Practical)
Final (Summative) Assessments (Written and Practical)
Professional Portfolio

A2.4 Mapping of Assessment Tools with Learning Outcomes

Below is a comparison of the suitable assessment tools against the learning outcome verbs used in this document

No	Tool	Learning Outcome Verbs
1	**Case Studies**	analyse; demonstrate; discuss; explain;
2	**Client Studies**	evaluate; list;
3	**Home Treatments**	evaluate; list; locate
4	**Blank Feet/Hand Diagrams to locate Reflex Points/Areas**	draw; locate; recall;
5	**Blank Diagrams of Body Parts to Labels A&P Items**	draw; locate; recall;
6	**2000 to 5000-word Assignments** At level 2 At level 3	analyse; assess; analyse; assess; critique, evaluate; synthesise;
7	**Interim (Formative) Assessments (Written)**	draw; locate; recall;
8	**Interim (Formative) Assessments (Practical)**	demonstrate; demonstrate understanding;
9	**Final (Summative) Assessments (Written)**	draw; locate; recall;
10	**Final (Summative) Assessments (Practical)**	demonstrate;
11	**Professional Portfolio**	analyse; articulate; assess; demonstrate; discuss; evaluate; explain; list; locate; recall; state
12	**Interview**	articulate, explain; list; recall; state;
13	**Project: Research based or audit**	analyse, design, evaluate, manage

A2.5 Client Studies, Case Studies and External Treatment Practice

A universal aspect of Reflexology (and other Complementary Medicine) learning is the Case/Client Study and Home Treatments. Performing treatments away from the training centre is vital. It enables the student to gain experience of a wide range of clinical conditions, develop confidence in dealing with people, strengthen conviction that reflexology *does* improve the potential for good health and *does* activate the body's own healing system to counter ill health.

The case study is of even greater importance educationally as it demonstrates the ability of students to **integrate theory into practice** and helps them **critically review** their progress. To students taking the academic route the case study becomes a tool to enable them to **evaluate** and **synthesise** their learning by producing an assignment around their practical experiences to **develop** and **refine** written communication skills.

A2.5.1 Client Studies

A Client Study is defined as '*a course of Reflexology treatment performed on a client during contact hours/clinic sessions **when the tutor/assessor is present** to assess the practical techniques being used by the student*'.

Unlike External Treatment Practice these will not be from the pool of family and friends that the student will gather for practice but should reflect the **real working environment** as closely as possible. Often these clients will be members of the public paying a reduced fee.

- A **minimum** of **three** client study treatments **per year** is needed to assess each student's practice. (In practice, when the policy of continuous assessment is followed, many more than three client studies will be observed.)
- **One** of these studies will be a **summative assessment** by an **external verifier/examiner** from the awarding/examining body (refer to section A4.2 in Appendix 4 – assessment guidance).
- The **second** of the three minimum client studies can best utilised as an **interim formative assessment** by an external verifier/examiner undertaken at a stage where the student has had time to develop sufficient skill and understanding to perform a treatment but also giving the assessor opportunity to deliver constructive feedback to both student and tutor prior to the summative assessment.
  To assess the widest range possible *the clients* for the three client study assessments *would be different people*. However, where this is not possible there is still merit in observing the evaluative and follow-up skills of a repeat treatment.

(A complete summative assessment must involve the assessor observing an entire treatment from consultation through to treatment recording and rebooking. This ideal would require a one-to-one ratio which may be rarely financially viable. Assessors will find providing constructive feedback at a ratio of more than three to one extremely difficult. However, usually the tutor will be the/an assessor and employing continuous assessment will enable the tutor/assessor to observe and assess all aspects of the treatment process albeit over a period of time.)

A2.5.2 Case Studies

A Case Study is defined as '*a course of Reflexology treatment performed outside contact hours/clinic sessions where **the tutor will not be there** to observe the practical skills of the student directly*'.

- **In the case of academic courses** these treatments will form the basis of an ongoing assignment over the minimum year duration of the course. The student will produce a **5,000-word** assignment **analysing** the treatment outcomes of at least **four case studies** (see A2.5.7 below).
- **In the case of vocational courses** these treatments will form the basis of individual studies covering **40** treatments. The student may choose to carry on case studies into a second year or start new ones

A2.5.3 External Treatment Practice or Home Treatments

Refers to all other correctly researched, performed, evaluated and recorded treatments that are not Client Studies or Case Studies.

A2.5.4 Total Treatment Requirement

One hundred (100) Treatments are required for the entire duration of training. This requirement alone may make the duration of the course longer than 1 year.

A2.5.5 Number of Clients for Case Studies

In a real working environment, clients may book a course of treatments or they may come just once. Many continue to come for many years. To reflect this, the number of individuals for Case Studies can vary from **Four (4) to 12 (12)** – the main criteria is the required minimum number of treatments for case studies – **40.** This will leave 60 home treatments to be recorded in addition over the entire duration of the course

A2.5.6 Case Studies (Vocational Courses)

Students will write up 40 treatments as case studies with an **introduction** to the client, **summarising** the treatments in the body of the text and ending with a **conclusion** noting the *effectiveness of the treatment and lessons learned*. (It may be that the number of the words involved in these write-ups may exceed 5,000 – it is the nature of the assessment that differentiates this text from the assignment for academic courses below.)

A2.5.7 Case Study Assignment (Academic Courses)

This 5,000-word assignment is designed to integrate the student's theory into practice by ensuring they reflect upon their treatments and the outcomes.

(Depending on the modular structure of the course this assignment may be in two parts – 2 × 2,000 words.)

They will compare and analyse treatments as the course progresses to decide upon the combination of **four sets of treatments** that will comprise their assignment. The choice of treatments to write up as case studies will be for the student and tutor to decide during their regular tutorials.

- One choice may be to compare four clients with similar health problems to **analyse** similarities to inform practice and **synthesise** new treatment regimes.
- Another combination could be **two case studies** with **minor ailments** to be measured against **two** more with **life-changing conditions**. This combination will help the student to 'demonstrate skill in different areas of activity and a wider range of contexts'.

Table A2.5 Examples of Case study, Client Study and External Treatment Practice combinations

Assessment	Client Studies Assessed 'in class'	Case studies Write-up assessed		External Tx Practice Records submitted/seen		Total treatments
Example 1 Vocational Course	3 clts × 1 tx = **3** Minimum practical assessment	4 clts × 10 txs 4 case studies written up	= **40**	10 clts × 6 txs	= **60**	**103**
Example 2 Vocational Course	2 clts × 2 txs = **4** 4 treatments assessed	6 clts × 6 txs 2 clts × 2 txs	= 36 = 4 = **40**	8 clts × 6 txs 2 clts × 5 txs 2 clts × 2 txs	= 48 = 10 = 2	
		8 case studies written up			60	**104**
Example 3 Academic Course	2 clts × 2 txs = **4** 4 treatments assessed	5 clts × 6 txs 1 clt × 9 txs 1 clt × 1 tx	= 30 = 9 = 1 = **40**	5 clts × 8 txs 1 clt × 19 txs 1 clts × 1 txs	= 40 = 19 = 1	
		5,000 word assignment			60	**104**
Example 4 Academic Course	6 clts × 1 txs = **6** 6 treatments assessed	2 clts × 10 txs 2clts with minor ailments 2 clts × 10 txs 2 × life-changing conditions 2 × 2,5000 word assignments	= 20 = 20 = **40**	5 clts × 8 txs 1 clt × 19 txs 1 clts × 1 txs	= 40 = 19 = 1 60	**106**

Note: 'Tx' is abbreviation for treatment; 'clt' means client.

APPENDIX 3

RECOMMENDED READING AND LISTS

A3.1 Reflexology Text Books

No	Author	Title	Publisher	Date	Place	ISBN
	Adamson, S Harris, E	The reflexology partnership	Kyle Cathie	1995	London	1-85626-149-2
	Bayly, D E	Reflexology today	Healing Arts Press	1982	Rochester, Vermont	0-89281-284-2
	Byers, D	Better health with foot reflexology	Ingham Publishing Inc	1983	Florida USA	1-891130-00-5
	Byers, D	Anatomy & reflexology helper areas study guide	Ingham Publishing Inc	1994	Florida USA	0-9611804-7-1
	Crane, B	Reflexology, the definitive practitioner's manual	Element/Harper Collins	1997	UK	1-86204-125-3
	Crane, B	Reflexology: an illustrated guide	Element/Harper Collins	1998	UK	1-86204-169-5
	Crane, B	Illustrated Elements of Reflexology	Thorsons	1998	London	0-00-715273-6
	Dougans, I	The complete illustrated guide to reflexology	Element Books	1996	Dorset	1-85230-874-5
	Dougans, I Ellis, S	Reflexology, foot massage for total health	Element Books	1991	Dorset	1-85203-218-6
	Enzer, S	Sole to Soul Reflexology	Soul to Soul Reflexology	1997	Australia	
	Gillanders, A	Reflexology a step by step guide	Gaia	1995	London	1-85675-081-7
	Gillanders, A	Reflexology – the theory and practice	Daniel	1986	Saffron Walden	
	Gore, A	Reflexology	Optima	1994	London	0-356-20992-X
	Grinsberg, A	Holistic reflexology	Thorsons	1989	London	1-85675-081-7
	Hall, N	Reflexology, a way to better health	Gill & Macmillan Ltd	1988	Dublin, Ireland	0-7171-3095-9
	Ingham, E	The original works of Eunice Ingham. Stories the feet can tell thru reflexology and stories the feet have told thru reflexology	Ingham Publishing Inc	1938	Florida USA	0-9611804-3-9
	Issel, C	Reflexology, art, science and history	New Frontier Publishing	1993	Sacramento, Ca	0-9625448-1-7
	James, A	Hands on reflexology	Hodder & Stoughton	2001	London	0-340-80397-5
	Kunz, K Kunz, B	Hand and foot reflexology – a self help guide	Prentice Hall Press	1987	New York	0-13-383571-5
	Kunz, K Kunz, B	The complete guide to foot reflexology	Thorsons	1984	London	0-7225-3915-0
	Lett, A	Reflex zone therapy for professionals	Churchill Livingstone	2000	Edinburgh	
	Mackareth, P & Tiran, D	Clinical reflexology, a guide for health professionals	Churchill Livingstone	2002	Edinburgh	0-443-07120-9

A3.1 Reflexology Text Books (contd)

No	Author	Title	Publisher	Date	Place	ISBN
	Marquardt, H	Reflexotherapy of the feet	Georg Thieme Verlag	2000	New York	0-86577-931-7
	Norman, L	The reflexology handbook	Piatkus	1996/ 2001	London	0 86188 886 3hbk 0 86188 912 6pb
	Pitman, V & Mackenzie, K	Reflexology, a practical approach	Nelson Thornes	1997	London	0-7487-2867-8
	Stormer, C	Reflexology – the definitive guide	Hodder & Stoughton	1996	London	
	Tanner, R	Step by step reflexology (5th edn)	Douglas Barry Publications	1990/ 2003	London	0-9540176-4-1
	Tanner, R	Reflexology the case history book	Douglas Barry Publications	1998	London	0-951 6203-4-7
	Tucker, L	An introductory guide to reflexology				1903348021

A3.2 Anatomy & Physiology/Human Biology Text Books

No	Author	Title	Publisher	Date	Place	ISBN
	Blakey, P	The muscle book	Bibliotek Books Ltd	1992	Stafford	1-873017-00-6
	Gray, H	Gray's anatomy	Parragon	2002	Bath	0-75257-431-0
	McMinn and Hutchings	A colour atlas of human anatomy	Wolf Medical Books			
	Plumley, JS	Surface anatomy. The anatomical basis of clinical examination	Churchill Livingstone			0-443-04084-2
	Smith, A	The human body	Dorland Kindersly	1997	London	0-7513-5271-3
	Solomon, EP Schmidt, R & Adragna, P	Human anatomy and physiology	Saunders	1990	Philadelphia	0-03-011914-6
	Tortorah, GJ Grabowski, SR	Principles of anatomy and physiology 8th edition	Harper & Collins	1996	USA	0-673-99355-8
	Tucker, L	An introductory guide to anatomy and physiology	Holistic Therapy Books	2000	Cambridge	1 903348 00 5
	Wilson, K Waugh, A	Ross and Wilson: anatomy and physiology in health and illness	Harcourt Publishers	2000	London	0-44305156-9
	Weston, T	Atlas of anatomy	Marshall Cavendish	2000	Singapore	981-232-3899

A3.3 Books related to Medicine – Conventional and CAM

No	Author	Title	Date	Place	Publisher	ISBN
	BMA	Guide to medicines and drugs	1992	London	Dorland Kindersley	0-86283-927-0
	BMA	British national formulary	*	London	BMA	0-85369-393-5
	Black	Black's medical dictionary				
	Kirby, J	Roxgurgh's common skin diseases	1986	London	HK Lewis & Co	0-7186-0472-5
	Dziemidko, Dr Helen E	The complete book of energy medicine			Gaia	1-85675-120-1
	Dorland	Dorland's medical dictionary (28th edn)		Philadelphia	Saunders	0-7216-5323-5
	Foundation for integrated medicine	Integrated healthcare – a way forward for the next five years	1997	London	FIM	1-85717-173-X
	House of Lords	Select committee on science and technology, sixth report on complementary and alternative medicine in the UK	2000	London	HMSO	
	Lorimer, D French, G West, C	Neal's common foot disorders, diagnosis and management	1997	New York	Churchill Livingstone	0-443-05258-1
	Mills, S Budd, S	Professional organisation of complementary and alternative medicine in the UK	2000	Exeter	Centre for complementary Health Studies. University of Exeter	0-9531757-1-5
	Oxford	Oxford Concise Colour Medical Dictionary	1996	Oxfordshire	Oxford University Press	0 19 280055 8
	Russo, H	Integrated healthcare: a guide to good practice	2000	London	FIM	0-9539453-0-8
	Vickers, A	Complementary medicine and disability	1993	London	Chapman and Hall	0-412-48690-3

*Bi-annual

A3.4 Other Useful, Interesting or Comparative texts

No	Author	Title	Publisher	Date	Place	ISBN
	Arnold, M	Chi reflexology, guidelines for the middle way	Moss Arnold	2000	Australia	
	Bloom, W	The endorphin effect	Piatkus	2001	London	0-7499-2132-3
	Booth, L	Vertical reflexology	Piatkus	2000	London	0-7499-2319-9
	Booth, L	Vertical Reflexology for Hands	Piatkus	2002	London	
	Breeding, D & P	Reflexology: success at the last resort	Breeding Publishing	1997	Florida, USA	0-9667577-0-X
	Brennan, B	Hands of light	Bantam			0553-345337-1
	Bryant, I	Foot massage and nerve tension	Kingsport Press	1978	Tennessee	
	Corvo, J	Joseph Corvo's zone therapy	Century	1990	London	0-7126-3868-7
	Enzer, S	Reflexology, a tool for midwives	S. Enzer	2000	Australia	0-9577215-0-1
	Enzer S	Maternity Reflexology Manual	Soul to Soul Reflexology	2004	England	0-9548060
	Fitzgerald. Bowers and White	Zone therapy	Health research		California	
	Ghalioungui, P	Magic and medicine in ancient Egypt	Stodder & Houghton	1993	London	
	Gooseman-Lrgger, A	Zone therapy using foot massage	CW Daniel	1988	Saffron Walden	0-85207-170-1
	Grinbergh, A	Foot analysis	Samuel Weiser Inc	1993	USA	0-87728-780-5
	Jora, J	Foot reflexology: a visual guide for self treatment	St Martins Press	1991	New York	0-312-05864-0
	Hall, N	Reflexology for women	Thorsons	1994	London	0-7225-2868-X
	Kaye, A Matchan, D	Reflexology – techniques of foot massage for health and fitness	Thorsons	1983	Northamptonshire	0-7225-0562-0
	Kunz, K Kunz, B	Hand reflexology workbook				
	Kunz, K Kunz, B	The parent's guide to reflexology				
	Kunz, K Kunz, B	Medical applications of reflexology				
	McTaggart, L	The field	Harper Collins	2001	Hammersmith	0-7225-3764-6
	Mochizuki	Zoku shin do: the art of east asian foot reflexology				

A3.4 Other Useful, Interesting or Comparative texts (contd)

No	Author	Title	Publisher	Date	Place	ISBN
	Somogyi, I	Reading toes: your feet as reflexions of your personality	C W Daniel & Company Ltd	1997	Cambridgeshire	0-85207-310-0
	Stormer, C	Language of the feet	Hodder & Stoughton	1995	London	0-340-64345-5
	Turgeon,M	Right brain, left brain reflexology:				
	Unwin, T Foulks, J	Reflexology, how it can help you	Cockatrice	1987	London	
	Wagner, F	Reflex zone massage – handbook of therapy & self help	Thorsons	1987	Northamptonshire	0-7225-1385-2
	Williamson, J	A Guide To Precision Reflexology	Quay Books	1999	Wiltshire	1-85642-176-7
	Wills, P	The reflexology manual	Headline	1996	London	0-7472-7822-9
	Seager, AM	Two feet from our thoughts, foot and nail conditions	Seager	2000	UK	0-913-7832-0-0
	Watkins Dr A	Mind-body medicine – a clinicians guide to psychoneuroimmunology	Churchill Livingstone	1997		

A3.5 Reflexology Forum Listed Foot (and Hand) Charts

No Name	UK Organisation	Book ref*	Date(s) devised	Where obtainable	Approximate cost and size		Hands Y/N
—	AoR	Reflexions; James A. Hands-on reflexology	2000	AoR Sales: Tel: 01379 676000	Feet	A1: £11.95; A3: £5.99	N
N Hall	BRA	Hall: Reflexology for women	1987	Bayly School of Reflexology Tel: 01886 821207	Feet	A1: £9.95; A4: £3.50	Y
B Crane	RS	Crane: Definitive guide	1989 (Foot); 1993 (Hand)	RS Tel: 01279 421682	Foot Hand	A2: £7.95 A1: £10.95	Y
B Coverdale	AOR accredited		1980	Naturecare Tel: 020 8699 0621	Hand and Feet	A3: £4.75; A2 £7.75; (Laminate) A2: £9.95	Y
A Gillanders	BSR/IGPP	Gillanders: Theory & practice		BSR Tel: 01279 429060	Feet	A1: £11.95	?
E Ingham/D Byers	IIR	Byers: Better Health with.....	1968/1984	IIR Tel: 01225 865899	Feet and hands pair	A1: £12.99; A4: 8.99	Y
C O'Hara	CaR	Mackareth/Tiran, Clinical reflexology...	1981/1996	CaR Tel: 0161225 9752	Feet and hands	A4: £3.95; A3: £6.95; A2:£10.95	Y
C. Stormer		Stormer: Reflexology – the definitive guide	1990	Pathwys School of Reflexology 01603 503794	Feet and hands		
R Tanner	IFR	Tanner: Step by step... (published by Douglas Barry Publications, London) ISBN 0-9516203-9-8	1973 (feet); 1996 (hand)	Douglas Barry Publications Sales: 020 7872 5745; IFR Tel: 020 8645 9134		£8.50	Y

*See Appendix 1

A3.6 Contraindications and Cautions to be Exercised in Reflexology

The list below represents conditions and situations that may occur. A rationale is provided. To ensure that all practitioners work within their limitation all areas must be covered as part of their initial training and an assessment made of their understanding of this area.

Condition	Contra-indication	Caution	Teaching point	Rationale
Acute undiagnosed pain		3	3	It is recommended that a client should be referred to their GP for a medical diagnosis of their condition. Clients are unlikely to attend with extreme pain – if it develops during treatment first aid training and emergency procedure applies.
Aids/HIV and hepatitis		3	3	These conditions should be covered during initial training which offers the practitioner an understanding of how reflexology can help such a client and when caution should be considered. Follow standard reflexology hygiene procedure.
Aneurysm – if known		3	3	Reflexology improves, not increases, circulation. There are no recordings of an aneurysm being precipitated, or immediately preceded, by reflexology, whereas many treatments will have been given, in retrospect, to patients unknowingly having an aneurysm.
Arthritis with inflammation or pain		3	3	Guidance during training to use appropriate pressure will accommodate client's needs.
Cancer-including blood and bone cancer		3	3	Understand the medical treatment and the likely reactions of treatment in relation to pressure. Awareness of low platelet count and potential bruising is important. *Working with people with cancer:* It is recommended that practitioners undertake further training and arrange supervision prior to treating in this sector to optimise support for the patient and themselves.
Cellulitis	3 (severe cases)	3	3	Be aware of the amount of pressure used; direct pressure on affected area is likely to be painful and therefore not appropriate. In severe cases it may be impossible to work the affected area at all. Using hand reflexology avoids contraindication.
Contagious or notifiable disease		3	3	**Any risk of infection and cross-infection** is a contraindication. The range of conditions is from the common cold and influenza to notifiable disease such as TB.
Diabetes		3	3	Appropriate pressure should be used as client's healing potential may be impaired, have lessened sensitivity (peripheral neuropathy), finer skin, bruise easily or be prone to ulceration on legs and feet. Regular treatment using lighter pressure will accommodate such concerns, may benefit the condition and facilitate monitoring of blood tests and condition of the feet (e.g. previously undetected *Gangrene* is contraindicated – see below).

A3.6 Contraindications and Cautions to be Exercised in Reflexology (contd)

Condition	Contra-indication	Caution	Teaching point	Rationale
Drugs or alcohol abuse – patient out of control or their mental state appears to be unstable	3 (if lacking the skills and facilities to cope)		3	If a client presents for treatment under the influence, there may be a risk to the safety of the practitioner. If a client who is dependent on alcohol or other substance, or is recovering, presents for treatment and is *not* under the influence; then the practitioner should be able to proceed with caution. Practitioners would be wise to arrange support or clinical supervision and undertake appropriate training. Risk of severe reaction/healing response. Some texts suggest alcoholic seizure is a risk.
Gangrene	3	3	3	Where a patient presents with undiagnosed gangrene immediate hospital attention is required, any delay increases the extent of surgery. Hand reflexology to ease stress may be an option whilst waiting for an ambulance. Hand and partial foot reflexology may be advantageous once the emergency is past which renders this a CI and a Caution situation.
Epilepsy		3	3	Have an understanding of the condition and how to assist and prevent injury in the event of a seizure – this should be part of regular first aid training.
Imminent medical tests or procedures	3 (depends on the test)		3	Dependent on the type of test being carried out and whether the client is having reflexology for the *first time* immediately before the test being carried out - the results might not be representative and medical overview may be distorted by the improvements resulting from reflexology treatment. As integration develops the monitoring of reflexology treatment prior to and during tests should confirm its effectiveness.
Injury to the feet		3	3	Practitioners should have been trained to adapt to all types of clients to accommodate their needs. Use hand reflexology or avoid affected area.
Heart condition, unstabilised		3	3	If a client is unstable then they are probably under the care of the hospital; treatment during this time would only be possible with consent, adequate supervision and the emergency facilities to hand.
Lymphoedema		3	3	National Guidelines state treatment should ideally be in conjunction with a Lymphoedema Specialist Nurse Practitioner. The option of treatment to the referral hand or foot (ie not of the affected limb) means this is not a contraindication. MLD techniques must not be used unless MLD qualified.
Medication		3	3	When, for a serious condition, the benefits resulting from reflexology might alter the amount of medication required, integration with the prescribing doctor is essential.
Menstruation		3	3	Some practitioners may chose to treat more cautiously if a client is prone to heavier flow or the reflex areas are tender, however, reflexology will usually help such a client.

A3.6 Contraindications and Cautions to be Exercised in Reflexology (contd)

Condition	Contra-indication	Caution	Teaching point	Rationale
Osteoporosis		3	3	Be aware of the fragility of the bones, use appropriate pressure and less vigorous relaxers.
Phlebitis		3	3	Be aware of the amount of pressure used; direct pressure on affected area is likely to be painful and therefore not appropriate. In severe cases it may indicate unstable DVT or be impossible to work affected area though unlikely on the feet. Use hand reflexology
Surgery		3	3	*Before surgery:* Practitioner could inform patient that a treatment may provoke a healing response - notably with the first treatment or patients who are very sick. *However,* the calming effect of reflexology can help to prepare for surgery and has been employed to replace pre-operative sedation. *After surgery:* Treatment can be very helpful post-operatively once signed off by, or with permission from, the surgeon.
Pregnancy		3	3	Practitioners should remember two lives are involved! Some practitioners may choose to avoid treatment. Some clients claim reflexology has helped during their entire pregnancy. Fear of litigation is often the deciding factor. *Working with clients who are pregnant:* It is recommended that practitioners undertake further training and clinical supervision to optimize patient and practitioner support.
Thrombosis/DVT*	3	3	3	**Reflexology improves, rather than increases, circulation. When the client is stabilised proceed with caution.** **After flying:** Check for signs of thrombosis, in some cases clients may prefer to defer treatment. However, the exercises suggested by airlines and medics closely resemble reflexology techniques and suggests reflexology be *indicated* rather than contraindicated.
Thyroidism, hyper and hypo			3	Client's medication may need to be adjusted in cooperation with their GP.
Varicose veins, severe		3	3	Skin may be delicate, direct pressure on affected area should be avoided.
Verrucae		3	3	Area should be covered or avoided and client referred for treatment. Use hand reflexology if there is extensive infection. Routine hygiene procedure will prevent cross infection to other parts of the feet, the practitioner and other clients.

*Condition may exist undetected and unknown to patient.
Remember it is an offence for therapists and practitioners to **advertise** that they treat the following: Diabetes, Tuberculosis, Cataracts, Glaucoma, Bright's disease (nephritis), Epilepsy, Paralysis, Locomotor Ataxy (one result of Tertiary syphilis) or Cancer.
One way of ensuring safe practice is to keep skills current. Ensure CPD hours are maintained or exceeded.

APPENDIX 4 NATIONAL OCCUPATION STANDARDS

A4.1 Mapping of Reflexology NOS against Core Curriculum

National Occupational Standards	Core Curriculum
Element R1.1	
Evaluate and process requests for reflexology	
Performance criteria	
(1) evaluate *requests*	13.1.1
(2) *communicate*	13.2
(3) obtain further relevant information	13.2.2
(4) explain clearly any fee structures	13.3.1
(5) establish any *particular requirements*	13.5.1–13.5.4
(6) evaluate requests	13.7
(7) make *arrangements*	
(8) explain clearly	
(9) record arrangements fully	
Range	
1 *Requests from*	13.2
2 *Communicate*	13.2.2
3 *Particular requirements*	13.5.2
4 *Priority*	13.3.1, 13.5
5 *Arrangements*	13.2, 13.5.1
6 *Unavoidable delays due to*	13.2
Element R1.2	
Agree the nature and purpose of assessments with clients	
Performance criteria	
(1) ensure the environment	13.1.1
(2) present an appropriate professional appearance	13.1.2
(3) ensure equipment, materials	13.1.1
(4) evaluate the client's initial approach	13.2.1
(5) introduce clients and companions	13.5
(6) throughout the process, communicate	13.7
(7) inform clients	
(8) identify clients' and companions' understanding	13.2.2
(9) encourage clients and companions to ask questions	
(10) only begin assessments when consent is obtained	13.2.3
Range	
1 *Work area*	13.1.1
2 *Initial approach and manner*	13.1.2
3 *Companions*	13.2, 13.2.3
4 *Confirmed in relation to*	13.2
5 *Communicate using*	13.2, 13.2.2
6 *Understanding in relation to*	13.3.1, 13.5.1
7 *Consent from*	13.2.3

(continued)

Element R1.3
Determine the nature and extent of clients' needs

Performance criteria

(1)	respect clients' privacy	11.7
(2)	conduct the assessment	12.5.1
(3)	support clients	13.1
(4)	contra-indications	13.1.1
(5)	observe aspects of the client's feet or hands	13.2
(6)	undertake examination	13.2.1–13.2.4
(7)	balance additional information	13.2.6
(8)	follow processes of reasoning	13.3.1
(9)	seek advice and support	13.4
(10)	halt assessments	13.4.2
(11)	inform the client	13.5
(12)	at the end of the assessment	13.5.1
(13)	make complete, accurate records	13.5.2
(14)	promote health and safety	13.7, 15.1, 15.2

Range

1	*Particular requirements*	13.5.1–13.5.4
2	*Aspects to explore*	13.2.2, 13.2.4, 13.5.1–13.5.1.4
3	*Observe in relation to*	13.1.1. 13.2, 13.2.1
4	*Aspects of the client's feet or hands*	13.2.1, 15.1, 15.2
5	*Client's condition in relation to*	Section 14, 15.1, 15.2
6	*Examination by*	13.2.1, 15.1, 15.2
7	*Conclusions in relation to*	13.2
8	*Complete*	13.7
9	*Records*	13.7

Element R1.4
Agree courses of action with clients following assessment

Performance criteria

(1)	communicate	13.1.1
(2)	explain the outcomes	13.2
(3)	base decisions	13.2.2
(4)	when necessary to refer	13.2.3
(5)	inform clients	13.2.6
(6)	record accurately	13.3.1–13.3.3
(7)	ensure any information	13.4.1, 13.5, 13.7

Range

1	*Communicate using*	13.1.2, 13.2.2
2	*Appropriate explanation*	13.2, 13.5.2 – 13.5.4, 15.1
3	*Subsequent action*	13.3.1, 13.4
4	*Level of risk in relation*	13.2.4 – 13.2.6,13.3.1
5	*Resources*	13.4.2
6	*Support by*	13.2, 13.3.2
7	*Completely*	13.7
8	*Interests of the client*	11.6.2, 13.2.3

(continued)

Element R2
Plan programmes of reflexology with clients

Performance criteria

(1)	ensure the developed profile	11.6.2
(2)	discuss the aims	13.1
(3)	agree staged goals	13.2
(4)	discuss and agree	13.2.1–13.2.6
(5)	discuss approaches	13.3.1
(6)	explain the possible effects	13.5–13.5.6
(7)	agree the location and timing	13.6.1
(8)	provide clients with information	13.7
(9)	clarify and confirm	
(10)	obtain the client's signature	

Range

1	Consent from	13.2.3
2	Companions	13.2, 13.3.1
3	Available and suitable options	13.5.2, 13.6

Element R2.2
Stimulate clients' reflex areas to promote the body's healing process

Performance criteria

(1)	ensure the *environment*	12.1–12.3
(2)	confirm *consent*	12.5
(3)	enable clients	13.1
(4)	throughout the treatment	13.1.1
(5)	apply appropriate *reflexology*	13.2.2
(6)	throughout the treatment	13.2.3
(7)	ensure the treatment	13.3
(8)	ensure the length	13.4
(9)	use alternative approaches	13.5
(10)	make appropriate adjustments	13.5.1
(11)	take the appropriate action	13.5.2
(12)	allow clients	13.5.5
(13)	offer advice	13.7
(14)	throughout the process	15.1
(15)	make accurate, legible	15.2

Range

1	*Environment*	13.1.1
2	*Consent from*	13.2.3
3	*Reflexology relaxation*	12.1
4	*Client's condition*	13.1.2, 13.2.6, Section 14, 15.1, 15.2
5	*Conditions*	15.1, 15.2

(continued)

Core Curriculum for Reflexology in the United Kingdom

Element R2.3
Enable clients to treat reflex areas for themselves

Performance criteria
(1)	justify requests	
(2)	clarify and agree	13.2
(3)	explain clearly	13.3.1
(4)	inform clients	
(5)	encourage clients	13.5
(6)	acknowledge the rights	13.6
(7)	respond promptly	13.6.1
(8)	encourage clients	13.7

Range
1	*Self-treatment*	13.6
2	*Potential responses*	13.3.1, 13.5.1, 13.6
3	*Effects*	13.6
4	*Client actions to take*	13.3.1, 13.5.1, 13.6

Element R2.4
Review the effectiveness of reflexology with clients

Performance criteria
(1)	actively encourage	11.6
(2)	discuss and review	11.6.2
(3)	actively encourage clients to offer their opinions	
(4)	offer the practitioner's views	13.1
(5)	offer sufficient time	13.2
(6)	reach agreement	13.2.2
(7)	where continued treatment	13.2.3
(8)	throughout the treatment	13.3.1
(9)	when the treatment	13.5.1
(10)	make accurate, legible records	13.6
(11)	compare the practitioner's knowledge	
(12)	if necessary, and with the client's consent	13.7

Range
(1)		Companions	11.6, 13.3.2
(2)		Outcomes	11.6, 13.3.2, 13.5.2
(3)		Opinions:	11.6, 13.7
	A	*Professional standards and codes of practice*	11.4, 13.1., 13.3. 13.4., 13.5, 13.6.3
	B	*Legislation*	13.2.3–13.2.5, 13.4.2
	C	*Employment and organisational policies practices*	13.1.1, 13.3.1, 13.3.2, 13.4
	D	*Communication and relationships*	13.2, 13.2.1 – 13.2.4
	E	*Work role and practice – reflecting and developing*	11.5, 11.7, 12.5, 13.1, 13.2, 13.3..3.2
	F	*Confidentiality*	13.2.3, 13.3.1
	G	*Consent*	11.4, 13.2, 13.2.3, 13.4.1, 13.4.2, 13.5.2
	H	*Anatomy and physiology*	Section 14
	I	*Health and social well-being*	15.1, 15.2
	J	*Illness and its treatment*	15.1, 15.2
	K	*The benefits, limitations and scope of reflexology*	15.1, 15.2
	L	*Reflexology principles and treatment methods*	15.1, 15.2
	M	*Practice management*	13.1, 13.2, 13.4, 13.7
	N	*Health, safety and the control of infection*	13.1, 13.4
	O	*Assessing clients' needs*	13.1, 13.2, 13.3
	P	*Assessing clients' needs in relation to reflexology*	13.3.1. 13.4, 13.5, 13.7
	Q	*Courses of action following assessment*	13.2, 13.2.2, 13.3.1, 13.3.2, 13.3.3
	R	*Planning programmes of reflexology*	11.6, 13.4, 13.6, 13.7
	S	*Reviewing the effectiveness of reflexology*	13.7

A4.2 Skills for Health Assessment Guidance

Below is reproduced an Assessment Guidance Document produced by Skills for Health July 2003

Quality Control on Assessment – Reflexology

This document will be subject to regular review to meet the needs of the sector and any changes in the sector and to ensure best practice assessment and verification processes and procedures are adopted and implemented.

The fundamental principles and beliefs relating to assessment of competence in Reflexology are:

1 A desire to ensure that consistent standards are achieved and maintained across all Awarding Bodies and training providers delivering reflexology practitioner training and qualifications
2 Assessment must be conducted by suitably qualified and experienced individuals who engage in relevant continuing professional development activities
3 The form of assessment of an individual's competence should be fit for purpose, i.e. it should be the most valid, reliable, fair and practical form of assessment for the knowledge, understanding and skills that are being assessed
4 Assessments should be carried out over a period of time and may be carried out simultaneously across two or more units
5 Assessments should be carried out in the workplace supplemented by assessments in realistic working environments to increase access to assessment. Achieving competence in a realistic working environment has to be seen as different from training and formative assessment (see additional paragraph on the use of realistic working environments)
6 There should be a range of assessment processes, tailored where acceptable, to meet individual needs taking account of prior learning and achievement
7 Well written and clearly defined National Occupational Standards and qualifications clearly linked to the National Occupational Standards establish a sector's benchmark of competent performance
8 National Occupational Standards together with clear evidence requirements and guidance to assessors on certain aspects of the standards provide the basis of consistent assessment practices
9. There should be equality of access to assessment to all candidates eligible to work in the occupational role that can provide evidence of the ability to perform to the National Occupational Standards. (Legislation may restrict practice)

Training is extremely important for individuals to develop the skill and abilities, and knowledge and understanding to fulfil the role of a reflexology practitioner. However, training is only part of the equation in establishing credible qualifications and methods of developing individuals.

Assessment is the key

Without some valid measure of achievement there is no way of being sure that all individuals completing their training have acquired the requisite skills, abilities, knowledge and understanding. The credibility of all training and qualifications usually is dependent on the quality of assessment and quality assurance procedures

National Occupational Standards

A set of mandatory National Occupational Standards has been developed for reflexology practitioners, which can be used as the basis for the development of training and qualifications. National Occupational Standards set out the activities that reflexology practitioners may be involved in. They identify the performance criteria i.e. what individuals must be able to do and the underpinning knowledge and understanding i.e. what individuals must know. National Occupational Standards that are suitable for use in continuing professional development are also available.

National Occupational Standards are useful to many different people and organisations – they can inform the development of training and training materials, they can assist with the development of job descriptions and with organisation development, they can be used as the basis for staff appraisals. They are often used as the basis for developing new qualifications and for mapping against existing qualifications.

Awarding Body

The Awarding Body(ies) for reflexology practitioner qualifications must demonstrate that they:

a) will develop and implement valid, reliable, practical and cost effective monitoring systems and quality assurance procedures

b) will consult with the Skills for Health Sector Skills Council on the development of Evidence Requirements to support the National Occupational Standards

c) will consult with the Skills for Health Sector Skills Council on the acceptability of training courses and qualifications for assessors

d) will consult with the Skills for Health Sector Skills Council on the development and refinement of technical and occupational criteria for the appointment of Verifiers/Moderators and Assessors

e) will comply with the guidance provided by the Skills for Health Sector Skills Council for the selection and appointment of the External Verifiers/Moderators

f) will liaise with the Skills for Health Sector Skills Council to develop a programme of professional development for the Verifiers/Moderators and Assessors

g) will provide the opportunity for External Verifiers/Moderators to participate in sector specific reviews and Awarding Body specific training events for continuous professional development on a regular basis

h) will liaise with the Skills for Health Sector Skills Council on the acceptability of any qualifications submitted by Assessors and Verifiers/Moderators as proof of their occupational competence other than any qualifications that can be approved at the launch of the qualification

It is expected that Awarding Bodies will ensure:

- the design of assessment practices does not discriminate between those taking full qualifications and individual units or groups of units

- that assessment instruments do not directly or indirectly discriminate against any particular group of people other than where legal restrictions apply

- where appropriate, suitable arrangements are in place for re-assessment of those areas where candidates have been shown to have 'not yet achieved'

- that the qualifications and occupational expertise requirements of all involved in the assessment and verification process will be regularly monitored and recorded.

Occupational Expertise of Assessors *(see Annexe A on the role of Assessors)*
Assessors for the qualifications must provide evidence of competence, which is defined as:

Holding/having held a position of reflexology practitioner for a minimum of **five years**. Their experience must be current to within the last **two years**.

This means that each assessor must be capable of carrying out the functions covered by the units they are assessing to the standards described within them, according to current sector practice

AND IDEALLY

Holding a suitable qualification in the vocational area. This is defined as:

A professional qualification in reflexology which has been externally validated by a recognised examining/awarding body and which meets as a minimum the National Occupational Standards.

OR

Assessment of prior experiential learning against the National Occupational Standards.

(The occupational expertise of assessors will be subject to amendment as additional qualifications become available, in which case, all assessors will be expected to hold a suitable qualification in reflexology.)

Assessors must have a full understanding of the National Occupational Standards (or the content of the qualification if NOS are not used) and requirements of the qualification being assessed; they must also understand the Awarding Body policies and procedures

All Assessors must either undertake approved training for their role as an Assessor OR must hold a recognised Assessor qualification prior to registration as an Assessor and prior to carrying out any Assessor duties.

Assessors must only assess in their acknowledged area of professional competence.

Assessors must be registered with their Approved Centre and be accountable to that organisation for their assessment practice

Assessors must demonstrate a commitment to uphold the integrity of the qualification and of the National Occupational Standards and their assessment practices

Assessors must be prepared to participate in continued professional development of their assessment skills

Assessors must provide evidence of maintaining professional competence. Assessors must be able to demonstrate to their Awarding Body that they engage in appropriate continuing professional development activities as recommended by the Reflexology Forum. The Reflexology Forum, in this instance, is acting in an interim capacity until the Regulatory Body for Reflexology is established

Internal Verifiers *(see Annexe A on the role of Internal Verifiers)*
Internal Verifiers must have a full understanding of the Reflexology National Occupational Standards and they will preferably hold an appropriate professional qualification in reflexology

AND IDEALLY

Internal Verifiers will hold/have held a position of reflexology practitioner for a minimum of **five years**. This experience should be current to within the last **two years**

Internal Verifiers will ideally have held the role of assessor, in reflexology or an approved and related discipline, for a minimum of **two years**.

Internal Verifiers must be in a position to contribute to and influence an Approved Centre's assessment policy and give constructive feedback on the way in which the policy operates in practice. They should be EITHER:

* employed by the same organisation as the Assessors OR
* accountable to the Approved Centre and have access to the evidence used by the Assessors

All Internal Verifiers must either undertake approved training for their role as an Internal Verifier OR must hold a recognised Internal Verifier qualification prior to registration as an Internal Verifier and prior to carrying out any Internal Verifier duties

Internal Verifiers must have a full understanding of the qualification requirements for the assessments they are verifying. They must also understand the assessment processes and Awarding Body policies and procedures

Internal Verifiers must demonstrate a commitment to uphold the integrity of the qualification and of the National Occupational Standards and their assessment and verification practices

Internal Verifiers must be prepared to participate in continued professional development of their verification practice

Internal Verifiers must provide evidence of maintaining professional competence. They must be able to demonstrate to their Awarding Body that they engage in appropriate continuing professional development activities as indicated by the Reflexology Forum. The Reflexology Forum, in this instance, is acting in an interim capacity until the Regulatory Body for Reflexology is established

External Verifiers *(see Annexe A on the role of the External Verifiers)*
External Verifiers must have at least **five years** practitioner experience in reflexology or a related discipline. This experience should be current i.e. **gained within a two year period prior** to beginning to externally verify

External Verifiers must either undertake approved training for their role as an External Verifier OR must hold a recognised External Verifier qualification prior to registration as an External Verifier and prior to carrying out any External Verifier duties

External Verifiers must demonstrate a commitment to uphold the integrity of the qualification and of the National Occupational Standards and their assessment and verification practices

External Verifiers must be prepared to participate in continued professional development of their verification practice

External Verifiers must demonstrate their ability to maintain credibility with the sector and to retain the confidence of the sector through commitment to ongoing professional development

Assessment

Candidates must be working on a **one to one** basis with their clients when they are assessed. **Assessments must also be conducted on a one to one basis with candidates**. These must include real clients **i.e. external/not known to the candidate/student** and may also include assessments in **realistic working environments**

A range of evidence sources may be used including observation, case studies/histories, professional discussion, written tests, presentation, professional learning log, tape/video, testimony. Evidence must cover a range of scenarios – **and at least one full assessed reflexology treatment must be included**. Because of the need to maintain **client confidentiality** assessment permission from the client must always be sought prior to assessment

Ideally **the final** assessed reflexology treatment **will be conducted by Assessors who have not been involved in the training and education of the candidate they are assessing**

No individual unit of competence should be assessed using only one form of assessment

Realistic working environments

A realistic working environment may be used to **support** judgements regarding competence in the assessment and treatment of clients. Clients may be drawn from colleagues or senior practitioners and they should be briefed to present a range of conditions not seen during assessments involving real clients:

- where the treatment is likely to be restricted to one session
- where it is likely that treatment will extend over a series of sessions where the client is returning for further treatment and review where the practitioner is not qualified to treat the client

The environment should enable the work activities to be conducted in **confidence** and meet the requirements laid down by the National Occupational Standards and professional bodies. To facilitate assessment, *audio and/or video taped evidence may be used* providing that permission has first been obtained from those involved

All assessments must be set up so as to replicate real work activities and the real working environment as closely as possible to those normally operating in the workplace. Realistic working environments are defined as:

- **Having a comprehensive range of demands, activities and constraints that are the same as/ very similar to those that would be met in a real work situation**
- Enabling candidates to access the normal facilities, support and advice that are the same/very similar to those that would be met in a real work situation.
- Putting candidates under time pressures, working demands and resource constraints that would normally apply in a real work situation

External Quality Control of Assessment

It is recommended that independent assessment is achieved through use of standardised case studies which would be submitted to the Awarding Body(ies) for external marking

In addition to the use of standardised case studies it is recommended that Awarding Bodies establish effective statistical monitoring systems to provide information on the performance of centres, assessors and internal verifiers over time. Awarding Bodies should use the results of this monitoring to inform the deployment of external verification and training and development events. Risk rating approaches should also be used to identify and evaluate the likely risks that assessment decisions may be unsound, so that external verification can be targeted effectively and prompt and effective actions taken to achieve reliable, valid and consistent assessment decisions

Effective **use of statistical monitoring and risk rating is dependant upon** the quality and quantity of data obtained. External verification procedures should ensure representative sampling of assessment processes and decisions, particular attention should be given to the final assessed reflexology treatment, and internal verification processes and decisions, as well as monitoring other key performance indicators in relation to centre performance e.g. planning, equal opportunities, resourcing, record keeping etc

Annexe A

The role of the Assessor

Assessors are responsible and accountable for:
- managing the system of assessment from assessment planning through to making and recording assessment decisions as required by the awarding body;
- assessing evidence of candidate competence against the National Occupational Standards within the qualification;
- ensuring the validity, authenticity and sufficiency of evidence produced by candidates;
- maintaining accurate and verifiable candidate assessment and achievement records as required by the awarding body.

The role of the Internal Verifier

Internal Verifiers are responsible and accountable for:
- regularly sampling evidence of assessment decisions made by all assessors across all aspects of the assessments in order to monitor, and ensure, consistency in the interpretation and application of standards within the centre. Sampling must include direct observation of assessment practice;
- maintaining up-to-date records of internal verification and sampling activity and ensuring that these are available for the purposes of external verification;
- establishing procedures to develop a common interpretation of the National Occupational Standards between assessors;
- monitoring and supporting the work of assessors within the centre;
- facilitating appropriate staff development and training for assessors;
- providing feedback to the external verifier on the effectiveness of assessment;
- ensuring that any corrective actions required by the awarding body are implemented within agreed timescales

The role of the External Verifier

External Verifiers are responsible and accountable for:
- visiting centres to monitor the quality and consistency of assessment practices and procedures against the National Occupational Standards contained within the award;
- providing feedback to the awarding body on the performance of its centres in maintaining the consistent application of the National Occupational Standards;
- providing assurance to the awarding body that approved centres are continuing to operate in accordance with the requirements of the approved centre criteria;
- recommending to the awarding body the imposition of an appropriate sanction or penalty, in cases where a centre is failing to comply with the requirements of the approved centre criteria. Awarding bodies must monitor the consistency of external verifiers in applying sanctions and penalties.

A4.3 Career Progression in Reflexology
(PoWFIH Jan 2003)

PoWFIH Career Progression Flowchart

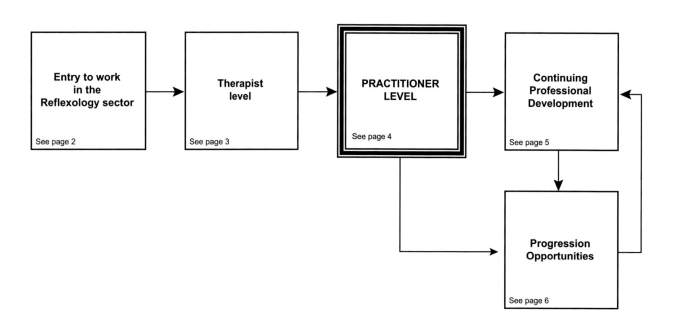

Reflexology Therapist

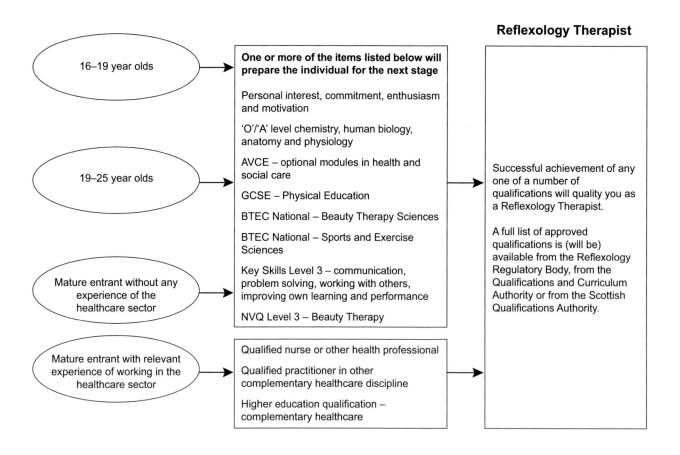

APPENDIX 5 CURRENT LEGISLATION

(Relative to Section 6 – Clinical Practice)

1. Employers Liability 1969
2. Social Services Act 1970 (Section 7)
3. The Fire Precautions Act 1971
4. Trades Description Act 1972
5. Health and Safety at Work Act 1974
6. Race Relations Act 1976
7. The Health and Safety (First aid) 1981
8. Local Government (Miscellaneous Provisions) Act 1982
9. Medical Act 1983
10. Data Protection Act 1984
11. Sex Discrimination Act 1986
12. Children Act 1989
13. Performing Rights (under Copyright Designs and Patents) Act 1988
14. Electricity at Work 1989
15. The Environmental Protection Act 1990
16. Personal Protective Equipment 1992
17. The Provision and use of Work Equipment 1992
18. The Work Place Regulations (Health Safety and Welfare) 1992
19. The Sale and Supply of Goods Act 1994
20. VAT Act 1994
21. Reporting Injuries, Diseases and Dangerous Occurrences [RIDDOR] 1995
22. The Disability Discrimination Act 1995
23. Sex Offenders Act 1997
24. The Fire Precautions (Workplace) Regulations 1997
25. The Working Time Regulations 1998
26. Crime and Disorder Act 1998
27. ECHR (Human Rights Act) 1998
28. Control of Substance Hazardous to Health Regulations [COSHH] 1999
29. The Management of Health and Safety at Work 1999
30. Protection of Children Act 1999
31. Youth Justice and Criminal Evidence Act 1999
32. Dangerous substances and Preparations (nickel) 2000
33. Care Standards Act 2000
34. The Children (leaving care) Act 2000

Students should also:

1. Determine any relevant **Local Authority Licensing Regulations**
2. Recognise Industry Codes of Ethics and Practice
3. Obtain and examine Codes of Ethics and Practice of any Professional Body they intend to join

APPENDIX 6 LEVELS

A6.1 Training and Education Levels

Since receiving its commission in July 2001 the Reflexology Forum Education and Training group has sought to prepare a curriculum that could bridge any perceived divide between academic education and learning and competence based, vocational skills training. This curriculum content has been provided equally successfully in University (Higher Education) and College of Further Education (FE) settings.

Historically, the bulk of training has been in the private school environment and this core curriculum will continue to be provided here.

The policy of the Reflexology Forum Education and Training group is to encourage the provision of funding to this important area of training, as often these are centres of excellence with smaller student/teacher ratios.

The situation regarding levels can be confusing to the lay person and no doubt this is not helped by the fact that there is confusion of levels within education itself. This affects the public as clients who may seek to ascertain the qualification of their reflexology practitioner or as potential students looking for a training provider.

A6.1.1 Academic Levels

These broadly relate to the three years associated with a typical university degree and have related outcome descriptor words that indicate the level of academic qualities required. Reflexology is a practical skill, but to practise effectively a sound theoretical base is required. Studying the science involved at an academic institution has advantages and should certainly not be viewed as impractical.

Table A6.1 represents a much simplified relationship of 3 educational models* reflecting the relationship of 6 levels of learning, 5 levels of experiential achievement and 5 levels of clinical practice demonstrating the integration of theory into practice.

Table A6.1: Academic levels and descriptors

| Academic level | Descriptors | | |
	Bloom's taxonomy	Experiential taxonomy	Benner's Spiral
1. Certificate I	Knowledge	Exposure	Novice
	Understanding	Participation	Advanced beginner
	Application	Identification	Competent
2. Diploma	Analysis	Internalisation	Proficient
3. Degree	Synthesis Evaluation	Dissemination	Expert

* Bloom (1956), Steinaker & Bell (1979), Benner (1984)

A6.2 Vocational Levels

These are levels designed to describe competence of practical skills as outlined on the NVQ framework. A comparison of Tables A6.1 and A6.2 will reveal that the academic level 3 does not equate with the vocational level 3 as they describe different things.

It is also apparent that a Diploma at level 3 does not necessarily equate with an academic (level 2) Diploma. This situation is not good for the reflexology practitioner/therapist who holds a Diploma or the client who wishes to rely on the skill that it is supposed to reflect. It is this disparity and confusion that this core curriculum seeks to address.

A6.3 The Recommended Level of this Core Curriculum

Those Universities that currently offer Reflexology modules do so at Academic Levels 2 and 3. Many are parts of Foundation Degrees in Complementary Medicine or Health Studies sometimes these courses are modules as part of a Nursing Degree where the level 1 is accredited to the basic nurse training. The *diploma* level 2 gives the student the ability to study and learn to practice reflexology **proficiently** (safely and effectively) with the required **analysis** and **internalisation** reflected in the assignments produced. The level 3 progresses the practice to **expert** level with the **synthesis, evaluation** and **dissemination** evident in the more extensive and rigorously marked assignment that often contains a research or audit element. The proposal of the Reflexology Forum Education and Training group is:

A6.3.1 The Recommended *Academic Level* of this Core Curriculum

- The first year of training will be at Academic, Diploma Level 2
- Where training providers can extend into a second year of training this can be at

   Academic, Diploma Level 2 or Academic Level 3

   depending upon whether there is a research element involved and the marking/ assessment criteria applied.

A6.3.2 The Recommended *Vocational Level* of this Core Curriculum

The rationale for this is that the NVQ descriptors for level 4 define most accurately a reflexology practitioner, the operative words being: 'Competence that involves the *application of knowledge and skills* in a *broad range* of *complex technical or professional* work activities performed in a *wide variety of contexts*. At this level the individual:

- must have a substantial degree of personal responsibility and autonomy
- is *often responsible for the work of others*
- is *often responsible for the allocation of resources*.

A graduate who sets up as a mobile practitioner or within a clinic setting needs to be taught the *application of knowledge and skills* in a *broad range* of *complex technical or professional* in a *wide variety of contexts*. In running their own practice such a person needs:

- a *degree of personal responsibility and autonomy*
- is *often responsible for the work of others*
- is *often responsible for the allocation of resources'*

The research or audit portion of the curriculum further argues that the course be at level 4

However, it is likely that as there is no precedent for level 4, the QCA will insist that this curriculum be presented at Vocational level 3.

Table A6.2: National Vocational Qualification level descriptors

The level descriptors are intended to be:
- **Indicative rather than prescriptive**
- **Used as an aid to the development of NOS and qualifications**

Levels apply to the whole of a qualification, although in certain cases (e.g. Key Skills and National Language standards) the levels can apply to units/standards.

Levels go up in complexity of activities, personal autonomy an for control of others/allocation of resources

Level 5
Competence that involves the application of skills and a significant range of fundamental principles across a wide and often unpredictable variety of contexts. At this level:
- the individual must have a very substantial degree of personal responsibility and autonomy
- the individual often has a significant responsibility for the work of others
- the allocation of substantial resources features strongly

Personal accountability for analysis and diagnosis, design, planning, execution and valuation feature strongly

Level 4
Competence that involves the application of knowledge and skills in a broad range of complex technical or professional work activities performed in a wide variety of contexts. At this level the individual:
- must have a substantial degree of personal responsibility and autonomy
- is often responsible for the work of others
- is often responsible for the allocation of resources

Level 3
Competence that involves the application of knowledge and skills in a broad range of varied work activities performed in a wide variety of contexts. At this level:
- most activities should be complex or non routine
- there should be considerable individual responsibility and autonomy
- control and guidance of others is often required

Level 2
Competence that involves the application of knowledge and skills in a significant range of varied work activities performed in a variety of contexts. At this level:
- there must be activities that are complex or non routine
- there must be, some-individual responsibility and autonomy
- collaboration with others, or membership of a work group or team, may be required

Level 1
Competence that involves the application of knowledge and skills in the performance of a range of varied work activities, most of which are routine and predictable.

APPENDIX 7 GLOSSARY OF TERMS

A&E	Accident and Emergency – department in hospital, also referred to as 'Casualty'
Allopathic	*medicine*. The usual method of treating disease, by inducing a condition different from the cause of the disease. A term that has become used to describe conventional, orthodox or 'Western' medicine. Cf Homeopathy
Alternative medicine	A line of treatment chosen or administered instead of orthodox, conventional or allopathic treatment
Analyse	*vb* to examine in detail in order to discover meaning.
Analysis	*n* the division of a physical or abstract whole into its constituent parts to examine or determine their relationship.
BCMA	British Complementary Medicine Association
CAM	Complementary and Alternative Medicine
Case Study	A course of Reflexology treatment performed outside contact hours/clinic sessions where the tutor/assessor is not be there
Caution	Any situation or condition, especially one of disease which demands more than the usual amount of caution when delivering a particular line of treatment
Client Study	A course of reflexology treatment performed on a client during contact hours/clinic sessions when the tutor/assessor is present
Clinical Reflexology	A designation used to indicate that the reflexologist practitioner has received training that enables him/her to apply safe and effective reflexology techniques to a broad range of clients and adapt the treatment to a wide range of clinical conditions with which clients may present
Complementary	Forming a satisfactory or balanced whole
Complementary medicine	1. Treatment of the complete (full complement of the) person including their physical, mental, spiritual and emotional aspects (ICM 1976)

2. Treatment (usually, but not necessarily holistic) that can be delivered alongside (complementary to) orthodox, conventional or allopathic medicine either with beneficial interaction or without conflict. [NB Definition 2 has become the more commonly accepted definition of this term] |
| **Contraindication** | Any situation or condition, especially one of disease which renders a particular line of treatment unwise or even improper. |
| **Counselling** | A process where a person in an understanding atmosphere enables another by purposeful conversation to make his own decisions given the choices available to him |
| **Diagnosis** | 1. *in medicine*: The recognising, via symptoms, the true nature of disease.

2. *in general*: Thorough analysis of facts or problems to gain understanding |
| **Evaluate** | To ascertain, judge, assess or set the worth or value of |
| **External Treatment Practice** | Or Home Treatments – refers to all other correctly researched, performed, evaluated and recorded treatments that are not Client Studies or Case Studies |

FIM	Foundation for Integrated Medicine – the former name of the organisation promoted by His Royal Highness the Prince of Wales. See PoWFIH
Healthworks UK	The organisation responsible for training in the Health Sector replaced in 2002 when the Sector Skills Councils were formed by 'Skills for Health'
Holism	*in philosophy n* – the idea that the whole is greater than the sum of its parts
Holistic	*in medicine/healing ad j* – describing treatment that takes account of the whole person with its facets of physical, mental, spiritual and emotional health
Homeopathy	*Medicine* a method of treating disease by using small amounts of a substance that, in healthy persons, produces symptom similar to those of the disease being treated. Cf allopathy
Homeostatsis	The body's ability to maintain a steady metabolic equilibrium within narrow limits by compensating for disrupting changes
Homeodynamics	An attempt to more accurately define homeostasis by the introduction of the idea of dynamic compensation as opposed to a static state
Hypothesis (*pl* – ses)	A suggested explanation for a group of facts or phenomena, accepted as a basis for verification or likely to be true
ICM	The Institute for Complementary Medicine
Know	*vb* to be or feel certain about the truth or accuracy of (a fact etc)
Knowledge	*n* consciousness of or familiarity gained by experience or learning; erudition or informed learning. (Erudition – extensive scholarship; learning)
Neonate	
NOS	National Occupational Standards – for Reflexology published by Healthwork UK in 2002.
Plethora	Superfluity or excess; overabundance
PoWFIH	The Prince of Wales's Foundation for Integrated Health – formally 'FIM'
QCA	The Qualification and Curriculum Agency – responsible for managing the national framework of qualifications
Reflex/reflexes	Points or areas on (primarily) the feet and hands which correspond to areas on the body upon which the reflexologist will apply specific reflexology pressure techniques.
Reflexology Forum, the	The emerging regulatory body for reflexology, constituted in 2002 and comprising at September 2004 of ten reflexology membership organisations having more than 100 members of practicing reflexologists: AoR; BRA; CaR; IFR; IGPP; IIR; NIRI; PACT; RS; SIR
Reflexology Package, the	A designation referring to the various therapeutic features of a reflexology treatment which in addition to the techniques used can in combination contribute to its effectiveness: quality time spent; one to one; eye-contact; touch; non-invasive.
Self Help	The opportunity for, and instruction of, clients and their partners to use reflexology techniques upon themselves in addition to practitioner treatment
Skills for Health	The Sector Skills Council responsible for training and learning skills for the health sector which replaced Healthwork UK in 2002
Synergy	The concept that the various parts of a whole working together are greater than the sum of those parts – See holism
Understanding	The ability to relate a variety of facts together to enhance knowledge

APPENDIX 8

REFERENCES

Benner P. From novice to expert – excellence and power in clinical nursing practice. Menlow Park, CA. Addison-Wesley publishing. 1984

Bliss J, Bliss G. How does reflexology work? Theories on why it does work. On-line available: http://www.reflexcal.com.howto.4.HTML. 15th Feb 2000

Clinical Reflexology News issue 14. Client or patient? Manchester. CaR. 2004

Crane, B. Reflexology, the definitive practitioner's manual. Dorset. Element Books. 1997

Dorlands Medical Dictionary 28th edn. Philadelphia. Saunders. 1994

Dougans, I. The complete illustrated guide to reflexology. Dorset. Element Books. 1996

Foundation for Integrated Medicine. Integrated Healthcare – a way forward for the next five years? London. FIM. 1997

Frandsen P L. Why does reflexology work? – Is the explanation found in the embryo? Denmark. FDZ. 1998

Ghalioungui, P. Magic and medicine in ancient Egypt. Stodder & Houghton. 1963. London

House of Lord's Select Committee on Science and Technology. 6th Report on Complementary and Alternative Medicine. London. HMSO. 2000

Kunz K, Kunz B. The complete guide to foot reflexology. London. Thorsons. 1984

Kunz K, Kunz B. Groundbreaking research in acupuncture to impact reflexology. On-line: http://www.reflexology-research.com/howto.html. 9th Jan 1998

Mackereth P, Tiran D. Clinical reflexology a guide for health professionals. Edinburgh. Churchill Livingstone. 2002

Melzack R, and Wall P D. Pain mechanisms: a new theory. Science. 1965; 150:971–979

Mills S, Budd S. Professional organisation of complementary and alternative medicine in the United Kingdom. Exeter. Centre for Complementary Health Studies, University of Exeter. 2000

National Occupational Standards for Reflexology. London. Healthwork UK. 2002

Norman, L. The reflexology handbook – a complete guide. London. Piatkus. 1989

Reflexology Forum, The. EaT Report on reflexology education & training in the UK. Manchester. Reflexology Forum 2001

Precedents for two-year training/education (Reflexology Forum EaT Report 2001) *(from Section 3 page 7)*:

Academic:	(e.g. Salford University [current]; Manchester University [1994–2000])
Vocational:	(e.g. VTCT at Bury College:
	Year 1 C1080 level 3 Certificate in Reflexology Techniques
	Year 2 C1033 level 3 Diploma in Reflexology (2002))
Private Sector:	(e.g. CAR Reflexology Practitioner Diploma. Modules 1 and 2)